Heart: Beating to Breaking

Heart: Beating to Breaking

Jemison

First Printing, 2024

Look at us, Horace! Quite the journey,
wouldn't you say

Contents

Chapter 1

Introduction

The major cause of death worldwide is cardiovascular disease (CVD) with 17.0 million fatalities every year [1]. This equals a staggering proportion of 31% of the annual global deaths. Important risk factors are smoking, obesity, diabetes, and age[1], which affect developed countries such as the USA in particular [5]. The largest portion (85%) of CVD patients suffer from heart attacks and strokes, mandating research for reliable early diagnosis and treatment in this field. In this introductory chapter, I outline the cardiac structure and its function (Sec. 1.1) related to the mechanical implication of MI (Sec. 1.2). Possible cures, including the principle idea of engineered heart muscle (EHM), are presented in Sec. 1.3. This is followed by the formulation of the goals of my work and how it will contribute to a better understanding of MI treatment (Sec. 1.4).

1.1 Structure and Function of the Heart

The human heart, as depicted in Fig 1.1, comprises four chambers, right atrium and ventricle which are connected to the respiratory system, and the left atrium and ventricle supplying the rest of the body with oxygenated blood. To achieve this, a delicate interplay between the electrophysiology, hemodynamics, and structural mechanics of the valves and chambers is orchestrated on every beat of the heart. In this subsection I will explain how blood is pumped during a cardiac beating cycle, what role the myocardial architecture plays therein and how MI arises and disrupts cardiac performance. The focus is exclusively on the left ventricle (LV) as it is the strongest and largest cardiac chamber and responsible for the blood circulation through the body [6].

1.1.1 Myocardial Architecture

The heart wall consists of three different layers, namely the inner layer (endocardium), the middle layer (myocardium), and the outer layer (epicardium). Both, the endocardium and the epicardium are protective layers, which shield the myocardium against the ventricular blood, and the pericardium [6]. The main constituent of the heart, though, is the myocardium which is responsible for cardiac contraction and thus its pump function. The myocardium, as depicted in Fig. 1.2d, is organized in layers that are three to four cells thick and connected by a collagen network. This anisotropic myocardial architecture is responsible for the equally orthotropic mechanical response as detailed in Sec. 2.2.1.

Cardiac contraction proceeds almost instantaneously in a wringing manner which

[1]In the USA, on average, men experience their first myocardial infarction (MI) at the age of 65.6 and women at the age of 72 [5].

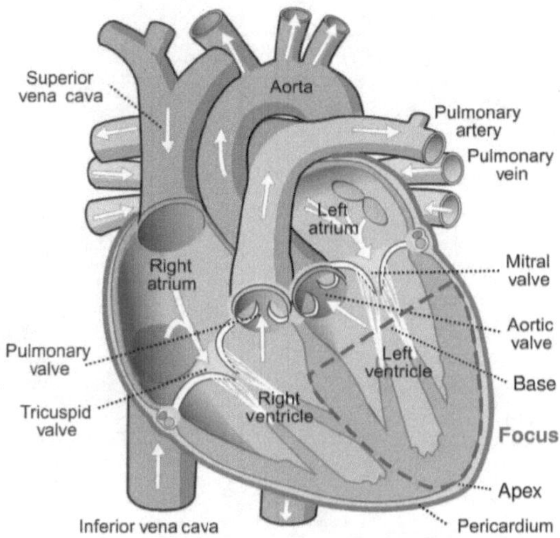

FIGURE 1.1: Schematic of the heart showing the atria and ventricles together with the flow of blood directed by the valves. As MI poses predominantly a threat to the left ventricle, the scope of this work lies in the highlighted focal region . Please note that neither the pericardium nor the papillary muscles attached to the mitral valve will be treated throughout this work. Image taken and adapted from Ref. [2] with permission.

not only compresses the interventricular cavity but also lifts the apex [7]. The reason for this is the helical arrangement the cardiomyocytes follow. As depicted in Fig. 1.2c muscle fibers coil clockwise at the subendocardium and counterclockwise at the subepicardium. Although, during contraction, this arrangement leads to a tug of war between outer and inner cardiomyocytes, the torque they exert depends on their distance from the ventricular centerline, favoring the cardiomyocytes at the subepicardium[2], leading to a clockwise contraction. A common hypothesis is that the twisting motion promotes sliding and shearing and thus rearrangement of the fibers, which leads to a magnified wall thickening, which in turn increases the pumped volume [8, 9].

1.1.2 Cardiac Cycle

The beating cycle of the LV is divided into a phase of passive filling (diastole) and a contraction phase (systole), during which blood gets ejected out of the heart. Starting with the closure of the aortic valve, as depicted in Fig. 1.3, the diastole begins and ends with the onset of contraction, which is accompanied by the opening of the mitral valve.

The stroke volume (SV) is an important measure of cardiac pump function. It is defined as the difference between end-diastolic volume (EDV) and end-systolic volume

[2]Additional residul strains amplify this effect (see Sec. 4.1).

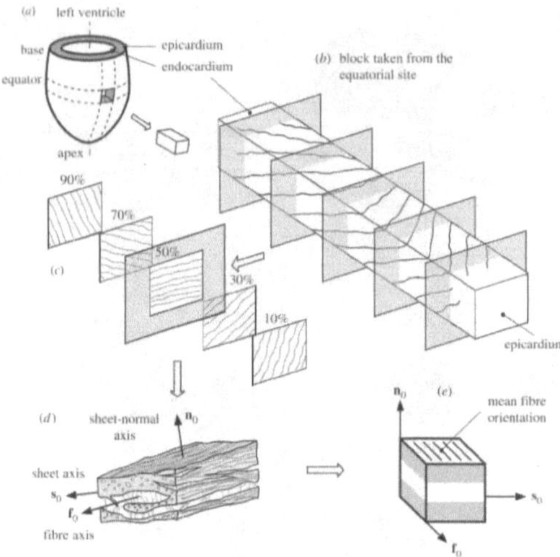

FIGURE 1.2: (a) Schematic of the myocardial architecture in the left ventricle. (b) Arrangement of myocardial sheets. (c) Transmural variation of fiber alignment. (d) Sheet structure. (e) schematic of (d) highlighting the local base system. Image taken from Ref. [6] with permission.

(ESV). Normalizing the SV by the EDV yields the so-called ejection fraction (EF)

$$\mathrm{EF} = \frac{\text{EDV-ESV}}{\text{EDV}}. \tag{1.1}$$

People with an EF of 50-70 % are typically considered healthy [10–12], while values between 41-49 % are borderline and an EF<40% may be evidence of heart failure or cardiomyopathy [3]. However, since several different physiological aspects factor into the EF, heart failure with preserved ejection fraction is a common condition (>50%) [13].

If a beating cycle features elevated end-diastolic pressure (EDP) while end-systolic pressure (ESP) remains constant, the additional volume gets pumped according to the *Frank-Starling mechanism* infamously referred to as "The heart pumps what it gets" [14, 15]. This mechanism presents itself as well on a subcellular level within the sarcomeres, which are the main building block of cardiac muscle cells (cardiomyocytes). Sarcomeres generate contractile forces through sliding exerted by myosin (motor protein) on actin filaments. Hence, the overlap of myosin with actin is crucial for the total force which is highlighted in Fig. 1.4. For large sarcomere extensions, this overlap is rather small and thus the motor protein cannot fully attach to the actin filament, wherefore contractile force increases as the muscle contracts. Once myosin binding is fully saturated, the length-tension curve plateaus until actin filaments get in contact with each other and myosin pushes against the so called z-disk. A typically linear decline in contractile force, determining the end-systolic pressure-volume relation (ESPVR), is the result [129, 16, 17].

Changing the ESP gives rise to a family of loops, as shown in Fig. 1.3. This is the so called ESPVR which is a robust measure of contractile performance (inotropy),

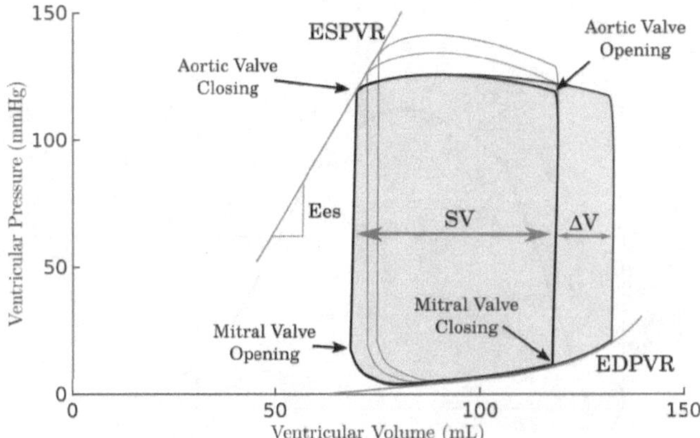

FIGURE 1.3: Illustration of the pressure-volume relation of the LV throughout an entire beating cycle. Closing of the aortic valve marks the onset of diastole, whereas systole begins with the closing of the mitral valve. Gray lines indicate the family of curves constituting the ESPVR which often times follows a linear relation (see Eq. 1.2) with the Ees being the slope. If the systolic pressure is kept constant while diastolic pressure rises, the excess blood, indicated by ΔV, is pumped according to the *Frank-Starling mechanism*. Colored areas highlight the energy consumption of the heart.

since it is relatively insensitive to ventricular pressure or beat rate, while greatly responsive to inotropic agents. Most often, the ESPVR follows, just as the tension of the sarcomeres, a linear relationship [18, 19]

$$\text{ESP} = \text{Ees} \cdot (\text{ESV} - V_0) \tag{1.2}$$

with end-systolic elastance (Ees) beeing the slope and abscissa V_0. The Ees spans a range of values 1-9 mmHg/mL as recorded in healthy humans by Refs. [10, 12, 20, 21].

1.2 Myocardial Infarction

Caused by plaques or thrombosis, ventricular arteries can become occluded, causing blood flow restriction. When a region of the heart becomes ischemic due to an insufficient supply of blood and hence oxygen, shortly afterwards the local tissue stops contracting during systole. Consequently, the tissue bulges under the immense pressure which is accompanied by a drop in pump function. If no immediate action is taken and this state lasts for too long, cardiomyocytes start to die over the next several days. This phase is followed by the onset of fibrosis which lasts for weeks to months, and finally the tissue remodels [24–26]. With fibrosis and maturation of the cardiac muscle tissue, it becomes stiffer initially, as shown in Fig. 1.6. This is due to collagen enrichment replacing the much softer cardiomyocytes and their alignment with the principle strain [27]. Constant stretching causes the material to thin out as demonstrated in Fig. 1.5, inducing a decrease of effective stiffness [23, 28], which, in turn, promotes bulging during systole. In addition, this effect increases the risk of

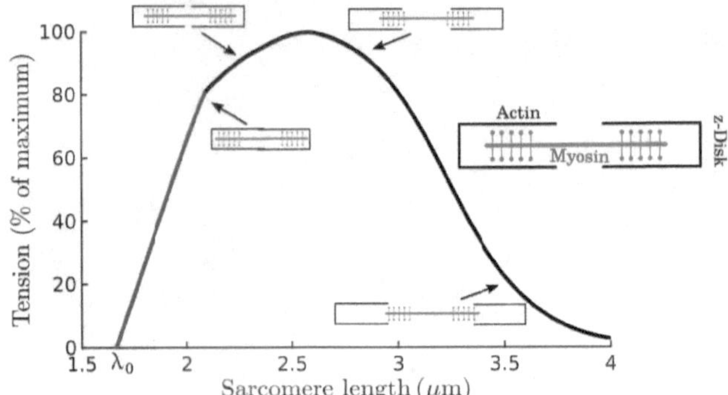

FIGURE 1.4: Sarcomere length-tension relation in cardiac muscles. The capacity to develop tension heavily depends on the overlap of actin filaments with the motor protein myosin and resistive counter forces once opposite binding regions get into contact [22]. The linear curve highlighted in dark red is most essential for the ESPVR, shown in Fig. 1.3. Parameter λ_0 is the smallest extension the sarcomere can achieve through contraction.

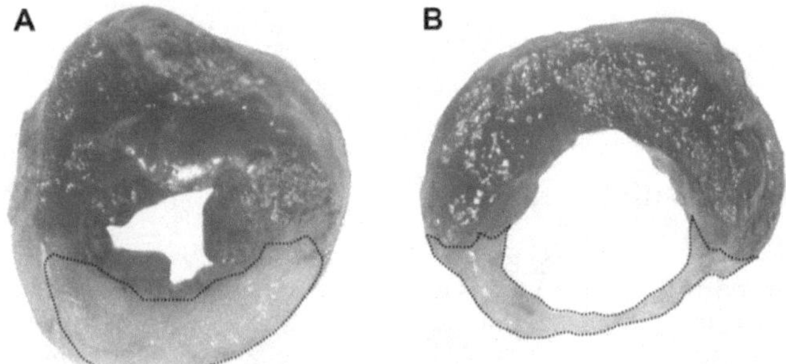

FIGURE 1.5: Infarct **A** 1 day and **B** 28 days after onset of MI in a rat heart. Infarct area is indicated using a dotted line. Wall thinning at the infarct site can lead to apparent softening of the ventricle (cf. Fig. 1.6) which promotes scar rupture. Image taken from Ref. [23] with permission.

scar rupture [29].

Implications for the previously introduced contractility indices are a decrease in V_0, which translates into a decrease in EF for constant EDP and ESP while the Ees stays constant [19]. Although a staggering proportion (∼50%) of heart failure patients does not suffer from a decrease in EF [21, 30], a linear relationship between infarct size and EF was reported by Refs. [31, 32].

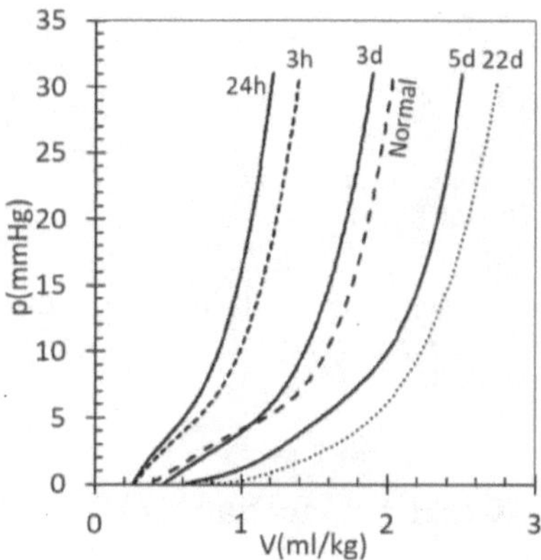

FIGURE 1.6: Impact of fibrosis and remodeling of the heart on the end-diastolic pressure volume relation (EDPVR). First, the material stiffens, but in later stages thinning of the infarct (see Fig. 1.5) causes apparent softening. Image taken from Ref. [24] with permission.

Myocardial remodeling often times entails infarct extension. It is a process of enlargement of the infarct and its border zone, progressively degenerating the LV and therefore increasing the risk of heart failure. Causes for infarct extension are still under current debate. For example, a decreased end-diastolic stretch in the border zone was found to correlate positively with infarct extension [33]. There exists also strong evidence that elevated systolic stresses in the border zone lead to a depressed contractile potential. This is followed by pathological cardiac growth associated with an amplified oxygen demand exceeding the marginal oxygen supply and therefore causing cell death [34, 130]. In consequence, MI treatment should not only aim at reestablishing initial contractile performance, but should also target lowered systolic border zone stresses.

1.3 Engineered Heart Muscle Tissue

Timely treatment of MI is crucial and potentially lifesaving. Especially reperfusion, as early as one hour after ischemia sets in, strongly benefits remodeling and viability of cardiomyocytes [24, 35] and can even fully reverse ischemia [25]. However, reperfusion is not always achieved and, instead, the condition becomes chronic. In such cases, injection of cells and synthetic extracellular matrices alike show the capacity to reduce border wall stresses, preserve scar thickness, and decrease scar fibrosis [36, 37]. Nonetheless, to this date, cardiac transplantation is considered the only efficacious treatment for patients with severe MI [38, 131].

The need for reduced diastolic stresses, together with the suppression of systolic bulging, likely necessitates cardiac remuscularization to achieve proper healing. A promising approach to accomplish this are patches made of EHM [36], as depicted in Fig. 1.7a. These EHM patches comprise embryonic or induced pluripotent stem cell-derived cardiomyocytes, collagen (type 1), and fibroblasts [39], mimicking healthy myocardial mechanical function. Depending on the maturation of the cardiomyocytes prior to implantation, these patches can develop contractile forces of roughly 25% of

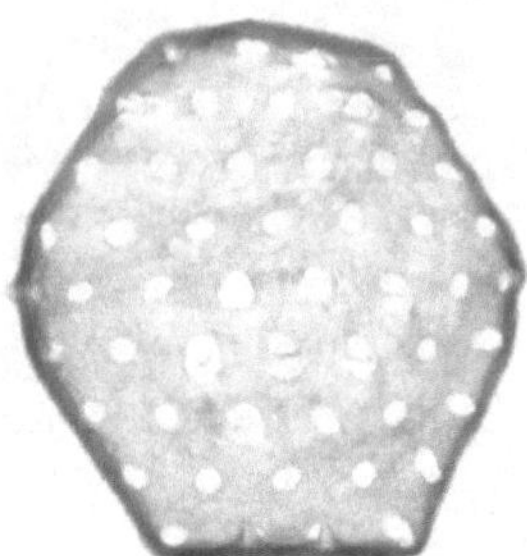

FIGURE 1.7: Hexagonal EHM patch used for implantation (received from *Malte Tiburcy*[3]).

those exerted by adult non-failing myocardium [40]. After implantation, the EHM tissue engrafts with the healthy tissue allowing strong vascularization which supports long-term cardiomyocyte survival and maturation [36, 41, 42].

1.4 Constitutive Modeling of Cardiac Mechanics

While the *ex vivo* mechanical properties of such EHM patches have been heavily investigated over the past two decades, its impact on ventricular dynamics remains unclear. Before implantation of an EHM patch, a few important questions must be addressed, such as:

- How much EHM tissue is needed?
- Where should it be placed and what geometry should it have?
- What micro structure, considering stiffness and fiber alignment, is most beneficial?

With the increase in computational power and improvement in numerical algorithms, in conjunction with advanced *in vivo* measurement techniques like magnetic resonance imaging (MRI), simulations further gain importance in cardiovascular research [43, 44]. The ability to change parameters, shapes, and functions individually allows for a broader and at the same time more detailed assessment of cardiac function and hence therapeutic factors. The increased interest in cardiac simulations over the last decades gave rise to a manifold of different models with varying levels of detail, ranging from passive hyperelastic modeling [6], to electrophysiology [45], to fluid structure interaction comprising hemodynamics [46]. Studying the effects of MI necessitates foremost a good understanding of the stress response of the myocardium, which facilitates patient risk stratification [47] together with contractile function [48].

With the aid of computer simulation, I aim to answer the questions above in a general, reductionistic manner thus elucidating the core principles for EHM patch design while, at the same time, laying the foundation for patient specific simulation of EHM treatment.

[3]Dr. med. Malte Tiburcy, Institute of Pharmacology and Toxicology, University Medical Center Göttingen.

In this work, I present the fundamental equations governing the structural mechanics of soft incompressible tissue in Ch. 2. This is accompanied by an exemplary spherical model of the LV explaining experimental data for the normalized EDPVR in Sec. 2.4. It follows an in-depth investigation of the influence of the fiber architecture in soft materials including dispersion of fiber orientation in Ch. 3, which comprises my publication [49] (see Sec. 3.2) introducing a novel class of mathematical models capturing fiber dispersion and its implications for numerical stability. In the subsequent Ch. 4 a ventricular model with healthy myocardium, infarcted tissue and EHM, successively is expanded, ranging from a transversely isotropic spherical model to an orthotropic, ellipsoidal model with realistic fiber distribution incorporating the findings and approach outlined in Ref. [49]. The influence of the EHM patch geometry and its fiber architecture are analyzed with regards to contractile performance and wall stresses.

Chapter 2

Structural Mechanics of Soft Tissues

Simulations of large scale deformations of soft biological tissue are founded on the mathematical concept of continuum mechanics. Its basics are shortly introduced in Sec. 2.1 and 2.2 and supplemented with an adaption to passive myocardium in Sec. 2.2.1. While, here, only the core features are laid out, the fundamental principles can be admired to great detail in the books of *Holzapfel* [50] and *Humphrey* [51]. The following Sec. 2.2.2 is concerned with primitive deformations frequently encountered in experimental assessment of elastic material properties. Sec. 2.2.3 focuses on incompressibility and how it can be approximated in numerical simulations. These simulations, throughout my work, are based on the finite element method (FEM) which is sketched in Sec. 2.3. This chapter, then, is closed with an application to real mammalian EDPVR data in the final Sec. 2.4.

2.1 Kinematics and Basic Definitions

When a body undergoes a deformation from state Ω_0 to Ω, as depicted in Fig. 2.1, the map

$$\begin{aligned} \Omega_0 &\to \Omega \\ \mathbf{X} &\mapsto \mathbf{x} = \chi(\mathbf{X}) \end{aligned} \tag{2.1}$$

is used to mediate between the reference and the new state. If the deformation is sufficiently smooth, it is said to be affine and the deformation gradient can be written as

$$\mathbf{F} = \frac{\partial \chi(\mathbf{X})}{\partial \mathbf{X}}. \tag{2.2}$$

The deformation gradient carries all geometric information necessary to describe a material's mechanical response. For example, it transforms any vector $\mathbf{V}$ from the reference configuration to the deformed state by mere matrix multiplication $\mathbf{v} = \mathbf{FV}$. The length of this vector is independent of rotations and translation, granting it the title of an invariant (or quasi-invariant). It can be written in the form

$$|\mathbf{v}|^2 = \mathbf{FV} \cdot \mathbf{FV} = \mathbf{F}^{\mathrm{T}}\mathbf{F} : \mathbf{V} \otimes \mathbf{V} = \mathbf{C} : \mathbf{V} \otimes \mathbf{V}, \tag{2.3}$$

where the right Cauchy-Green deformation tensor is introduced as

$$\mathbf{C} = \mathbf{F}^{\mathrm{T}}\mathbf{F}. \tag{2.4}$$

The orthotropic nature of myocardium, which is due to a clear distinction between fiber ($\mathbf{f}_0$), sheet ($\mathbf{s}_0$) and normal ($\mathbf{n}_0$) direction, forming an orthonormal base system, is demonstrated in Fig. 2.3. With the aim to address deformations in these distinct directions, the three invariants, based on Eq. 2.3,

$$I_{4f} = \mathbf{C} : \mathbf{f}_0 \otimes \mathbf{f}_0, \qquad I_{4s} = \mathbf{C} : \mathbf{s}_0 \otimes \mathbf{s}_0, \qquad \text{and} \qquad I_{4n} = \mathbf{C} : \mathbf{n}_0 \otimes \mathbf{n}_0 \tag{2.5}$$

are commonly used in the literature. The sum of the invariants given in Eq. 2.5 yields yet another invariant, which measures the length change of the diagonal of a cube spanned by the three base vectors

$$I_1 = \sum_{i \in \{\text{f,s,n}\}} I_{4i} = \mathbf{C} : \mathbb{I} = \text{tr}(\mathbf{C}), \tag{2.6}$$

where $\mathbb{I}$ refers to the identity matrix. These invariants prove their value in Sec. 2.2, where they are used to formulate an objective strain energy function, with "objective" meaning that the physics they describe does not change as the deformed body gets translated or rotated, thereby making them independent of the frame of observation.

Myocardium, however, is too complex to be described by these invariants alone, as it displays coupling between the different fibers it is comprised of. This connection can be taken into account by the mixing term

$$I_{8fs} = \mathbf{C} : \mathbf{f}_0 \otimes \mathbf{s}_0, \tag{2.7}$$

which measures the shear between fiber and sheet direction. For completeness, it should be mentioned, that, when dealing with the energy stored in a deformed body, it is oftentimes convenient to use a length measure associating zero stretch when the body is in its reference. Such a strain measure can be obtained by replacing the right Cauchy-Green with the Green-Lagrange strain tensor

$$\mathbf{E} = \frac{1}{2}(\mathbf{C} - \mathbb{I}) \tag{2.8}$$

in Eqs. 2.6 and 2.5. Both, the right Cauchy-Green, as well as the Green-Lagrange strain tensor are symmetric by design. Therefore gradients with respect to them exhibit an ambiguity in their definition [52]. For the applications in this work, it is important that the derivative of any given function ϕ with respect to a symmetric tensor $\mathbf{A}$ also is symmetric, wherefore we use the interpretation

$$\left(\frac{\partial \phi}{\partial \mathbf{A}}\right)_{\alpha\beta} = \frac{1}{2}\left(\frac{\partial \phi}{\partial A_{\alpha\beta}} + \frac{\partial \phi}{\partial A_{\beta\alpha}}\right) \tag{2.9}$$

Beyond length and shear measures, the deformation gradient also offers a measure of the local volume change with

$$J = \det(\mathbf{F}). \tag{2.10}$$

If $J > 1$ the body expanded, contrasting compression in which case $J < 1$. An incompressible material demands the constraint $J = 1$.

Knowing how volumes and vectors change under deformation, it is easy to derive how surface elements transform. Let $\mathbf{dx}$ be an arbitrary infinitesimal vector in the

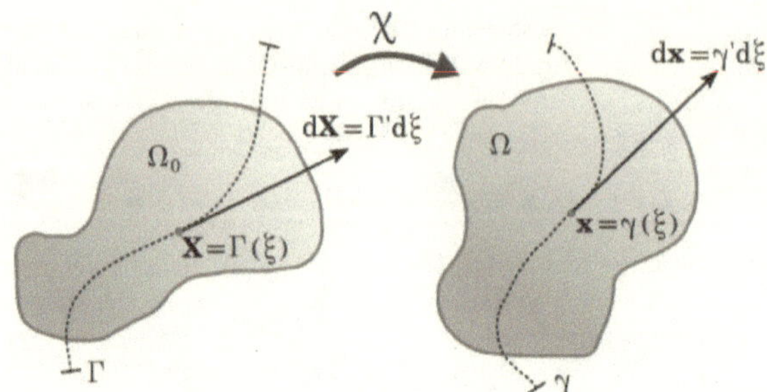

FIGURE 2.1: Deformation map χ, as defined in Eq. 2.1, transforms vector $\gamma' = \mathbf{F}\Gamma'$ according to Eq. 2.2.

deformed state, which, together with the surface element $\mathbf{ds}$, spans the volume

$$\begin{aligned} &\mathbf{ds} \cdot \mathbf{dx} = \mathrm{d}V = J\mathrm{d}V_0 \\ \Rightarrow\ &\mathbf{ds} \cdot \mathbf{dx} = J\mathbf{dS} \cdot \mathbf{dX} = J\mathbf{dS} \cdot \mathbf{F}^{-1}\mathbf{dx} = J\mathbf{F}^{-\mathrm{T}}\mathbf{dS} \cdot \mathbf{dx}, \end{aligned} \tag{2.11}$$

where $\mathbf{dX}$ is the corresponding vector and V_0 is the corresponding volume element in the reference configuration. Since the choice of $\mathbf{dx}$ was arbitrary, the equality

$$\mathbf{ds} = J\mathbf{F}^{-\mathrm{T}}\mathbf{dS}, \tag{2.12}$$

also known as *Nanson's formula*, is obtained.

2.2 Constitutive Modeling

When describing the forces developed by a deformed elastic body, this is done similarly as with classical, one-dimensional springs. The energy density Ψ depends on the deformation $\mathbf{F}$ (Eq. 2.2) through $\mathbf{C}$ (Eq. 2.4) and is measured per volume in the undeformed state. The force follows from the gradient of the energy density with respect to the performed deformation consequently. To arrive there, first, the true stress $\boldsymbol{\sigma}$ is introduced, which relates to the true force $\mathbf{dg}$ acting on a given infinitesimal surface element $\mathbf{ds}$ via

$$\mathbf{dg} = \boldsymbol{\sigma}\mathbf{ds}. \tag{2.13}$$

In the next step, it is shown how the total energy of the body

$$W = \int_{\Omega_0} \Psi \mathrm{d}V_0, \tag{2.14}$$

subject to externally driven infinitesimal deformation $\delta\mathbf{x}$, changes. With the same expressions as in Sec. 2.1 it follows that

$$\begin{aligned} \delta W &= \oint_{\partial\Omega} \delta\mathbf{x} \cdot \mathrm{d}\mathbf{g} \overset{Eq.2.13}{=} \oint_{\partial\Omega} \delta\mathbf{x} \cdot \boldsymbol{\sigma}\mathrm{d}\mathbf{s} \\ &\overset{Gauss-law}{=} \int_{\Omega} \mathrm{div}(\delta\mathbf{x} \cdot \boldsymbol{\sigma})\mathrm{d}V = \int_{\Omega} \mathrm{grad}(\delta\mathbf{x}) : \boldsymbol{\sigma} + \delta\mathbf{x} \cdot \cancelto{0}{\mathrm{div}\boldsymbol{\sigma}}\,\mathrm{d}V \\ &\overset{Chain-rule}{=} \int_{\Omega} \mathrm{Grad}(\delta\mathbf{x})\mathbf{F}^{-1} : \boldsymbol{\sigma}\mathrm{d}V = \int_{\Omega_0} (\delta\mathbf{F})\mathbf{F}^{-1} : \boldsymbol{\sigma} J \mathrm{d}V_0. \end{aligned} \tag{2.15}$$

Therein, div and grad refer to the divergence and gradient in the deformed state, while Grad refers to the gradient in the reference state. Since all internal forces have to cancel, it follows that divσ=0. Knowing that a given deformation does not touch the reference configuration, the variation and the integral commute, such that Eq. 2.14 yields

$$\delta W = \int_{\Omega_0} \delta\Psi \mathrm{d}V_0. \tag{2.16}$$

As this equality must hold for any arbitrary subdomain of Ω_0, it can, thus, be concluded that

$$\delta\Psi = J\boldsymbol{\sigma}\mathbf{F}^{-T} : \delta\mathbf{F} \qquad \Rightarrow \qquad \boldsymbol{\sigma} = J^{-1}\frac{\partial\Psi}{\partial\mathbf{F}}\mathbf{F}^{T}. \tag{2.17}$$

The tensor $\boldsymbol{\sigma}$ is also known as Cauchy stress. Similarly, other stress tensors can be defined, depending on which state the stress refers to. The first Piola-Kirchoff stress tensor, defined as

$$\mathbf{P} = \frac{\partial\Psi}{\partial\mathbf{F}} = J^{-1}\boldsymbol{\sigma}\mathbf{F}^{-T}, \tag{2.18}$$

relates the true forces given in Eq. 2.13 to the reference area via *Nanson's formula* (Eq. 2.12):

$$\mathrm{d}\mathbf{g} = \mathbf{P}\mathrm{d}\mathbf{S}. \tag{2.19}$$

In addition to the reference area, the second Piola-Kirchoff stress tensor also translates the forces into the reference configuration, thus reading

$$\mathbf{S} = \mathbf{F}^{-1}\mathbf{P} = \frac{\partial\Psi}{\partial\mathbf{E}}, \tag{2.20}$$

where the definition of $\mathbf{E}$ is given in Eq. 2.8.

To arrive at the expressions of stress in terms of the internal energy density Ψ, the equilibrium equation divσ=0 was used. For completeness, the nonequilibrium equation including external body forces $\mathbf{b}$, also known as *Cauchy's first equation of motion* [50], is presented:

$$\mathrm{div}\sigma + \mathbf{b} = \rho\mathbf{a}, \tag{2.21}$$

where ρ is the mass density and $\mathbf{a}$ its acceleration. This equation becomes important, for example, if gravitation and viscoelasticity are no longer negligible.

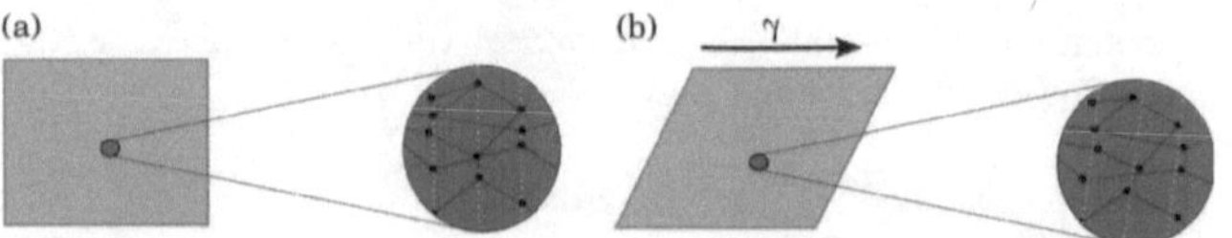

FIGURE 2.2: A schematic of an undeformed (a) and a deformed (b) fiber network undergoing non-affine shear. In case of an affine deformation the network nodes located along the dashed lines in (a), representing the far field deformation, would stay connected to it after deformation took place (c.f. Ref. [56]).

2.2.1 Passive Myocardium

With the ingredients introduced so far in this chapter, a huge plethora of different energy densities describing all kinds of soft (biological) tissues can be formulated, a great proportion of which are thoroughly reviewed in [53]. Another review, solely concerned with the description of orthotropic myocardium, is given by *Holzapfel & Ogden* [6]. After comparison of the already existing models, they propose an exponential energy density, termed Holzapfel-Ogden (HO) model given by

$$\Psi^{\mathrm{HO}} = \frac{a}{2b}\left(e^{b(I_1-3)} - 1\right) + \sum_{i=f,s} \frac{a_i}{2b_i}\left(e^{b_i(I_{4i}-1)^2} - 1\right) + \frac{a_{fs}}{2b_{fs}}\left(e^{b_{fs}I_{8fs}^2} - 1\right), \quad (2.22)$$

for which the invariants I_k, with $k \in \{1, 4s, 4f, 8fs\}$, can be looked up in Sec. 2.1 and the material parameters $a, b, a_f, b_f, a_s, b_s, a_{fs}$, and b_{fs} have to be matched with regards to a particular application. The individual summands are meant to represent the ground matrix, fibers, sheets, and interactions between fibers and sheets respectively. Employing such an additive superposition of different energy terms quietly postulates that the constituents do not interact with one another. This is, by all means, a strong simplification and evidently not valid on a microscopic scale where the polymer network gives rise to complex dynamics which cannot be captured by a simple mean field approach [54]. Another simplification, which is interwoven with the former, is introduced by the use of the macroscopic deformation regardless of the structure that is deformed. Polarized light imaging, however, unveils the discrepancy of the deformation between ground matrix and fibers in, for example, tendons [55]. When, on a microscopic level, the deformations of different constituents of a material are distinct and thus different from the far field as pictured in Fig. 2.2, the macroscopic deformation is said to be non-affine [56].

Despite all reservations, the HO model not only captures the experimental data displayed in Fig. 2.3 very nicely, its potency is also demonstrated in plenty other studies, including the aforementioned simple shear analysis [57, 58], patient specific heart modeling [59–61], and - after a small adaption - description of arterial walls [50, 62], making it a splendid candidate for cardiac mechanic modeling.

The Cauchy stress, adopted from Eq. 2.17, for the particular energy density given in Eq. 2.22 then reads

$$\begin{aligned}\boldsymbol{\sigma} =& a e^{b(I_1-3)}\mathbf{F}\mathbf{F}^{\mathrm{T}} + 2a_f(I_{4f}-1)e^{b_f(I_{4f}-1)^2}\mathbf{f}\otimes\mathbf{f} \\ &+ 2a_s(I_{4s}-1)e^{b_s(I_{4s}-1)^2}\mathbf{s}\otimes\mathbf{s} + a_{fs}I_{8fs}e^{b_{fs}I_{8fs}^2}(\mathbf{f}\otimes\mathbf{s}+\mathbf{s}\otimes\mathbf{f}),\end{aligned} \quad (2.23)$$

where $\mathbf{f} = \mathbf{F}\mathbf{f}_0$ and $\mathbf{s} = \mathbf{F}\mathbf{s}_0$ are used.

2.2.2 Basic Deformations

When experiments are conducted to obtain the material properties of soft biological tissue, there are several deformation protocols commonly utilized, namely pure shear, simple shear, monoaxial stretch, and biaxial stretch. To the best of my knowledge, there is currently no model that can capture adequately more than one of these protocols for the same cardiac tissue sample at once. Hence, which among these protocols to utilize depends on the application the data should be used for. For example, if the diastole is to be simulated, biaxial stretch tests are a promising candidate, since it most accurately captures the deformation emerging in the real heart, whereas strong shearing during systole might motivate the use of simple shear data instead. However, the lack of understanding of the interplay between these two deformation modes might nourishes the need for new experiments in the future.

One possible explanation for the lack of globally valid models may be that the experiments are not conducted in a transmissible fashion. The tissue patches for biaxial stretch tests typically have to be much larger than those for shear (25x25x2 mm *vs.* 4x4x4 mm), thus comprising a larger variety of fiber families. Tissue softening also comes into play, which rarely is captured in constitutive modeling but certainly will have different peculiarity for the various protocols. Further, compressible effects are differently pronounced in distinct experiments and lack a concise mathematical understanding, if they are even included at all.

Alternatively, it cannot be dismissed that likely myocardium is by far more complex in its nature than it can be captured by the few parameters - 8 in the case of the HO model - typically used. The macroscopic description shows deficiencies with regards to the entangled interactions of the different fiber families and cells [39].

Bearing that in mind, I further present mathematical descriptions for the two loading protocols that will be used as a reference for material properties throughout this work. In Fig. 2.3 a cube undergoing simple shear in the $(\mathbf{v}_1\mathbf{v}_2)$-plane is portrayed. The corresponding deformation gradients are given by

$$\mathbf{F} = \mathbb{I} + \gamma \mathbf{v}_i \otimes \mathbf{v}_j \tag{2.24}$$

with $(i, j) = (2, 1)$ if $\mathbf{v}_1$ is sheared with amplitude γ in $\mathbf{v}_2$ direction and $(i, j) = (1, 2)$ vice versa. Together with Eq. 2.22 it is now possible to capture the tissue mechanics as shown in Fig. 2.3 using a classical χ^2-Test . The same analysis also can be applied to biaxial stretch. In this case, the deformation gradient takes the form

$$\mathbf{F} = \gamma \mathbf{v}_i \otimes \mathbf{v}_i + \eta \mathbf{v}_j \otimes \mathbf{v}_j + \frac{1}{\gamma\eta} \mathbf{v}_k \otimes \mathbf{v}_k \tag{2.25}$$

where γ and η are the respective stretch amplitude. If the stretch ratio $\gamma/\eta = 1$ the protocol is also called equibiaxial stretch. Please note that for the description of both deformation gradients, one corresponding to simple shear and the other to biaxial stretch, the vectors $\mathbf{v}_\alpha$ with $\alpha \in \{i, j, k\}$ have to be orthonormal and typically correspond to the fiber, sheet, and normal direction introduced in Eq. 2.5. For experimental data of human cardiac tissue [57] the resultant optimized parameters can be found in Tab. 2.1.

2.2.3 Incompressibility

With Eq. 2.22 the tissue is treated as incompressible, an assumption that has to be reconsidered for two different reasons. First, experiments have shown significant changes in tissue volume related to fluid flow through the vascular system. The total

	a (kPa)	b	$a_f\,(kPa)$	b_f	a_s (kPa)	b_s	$a_{fs}\,(kPa)$	b_{fs}
Simple Shear	0.945	6.93	3.51	18.3	0.0942	54.3	0.338	1.58
Biaxial Stretch	1.025	22.8	0.985	42.2	—	—	—	—

TABLE 2.1: Best fit parameters obtained from a gradient based χ^2-test for the HO model to experimental human data depicted in Fig. 2.3. Nonlinear coefficients b and b_f are strongly pronounced in the biaxial data set. Due to a deficit in independence of the different biaxial modes, which is discussed in Ref. [63], terms belonging to a_s and a_{fs} are discarded in this case.

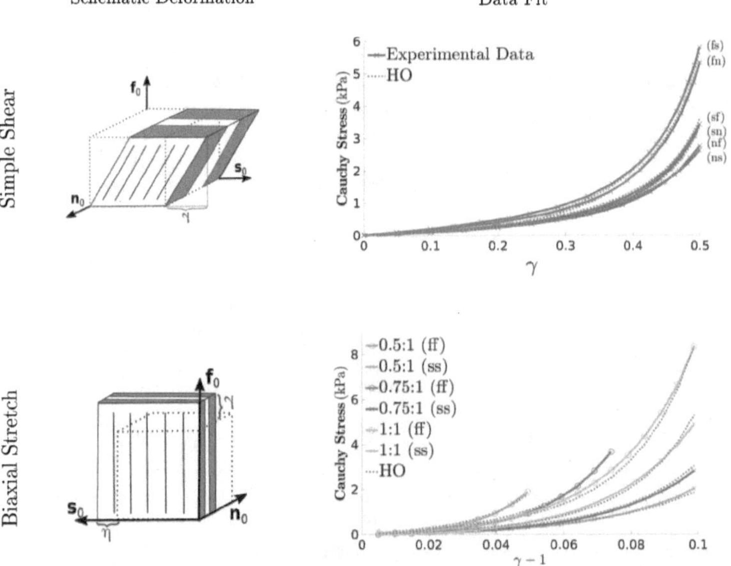

FIGURE 2.3: Left column: Schematic of the different deformation protocols according to Eq. 2.24 and 2.25. Right Column: Corresponding experimental human cardiac data taken from Ref. [57] together with the result of the least χ^2-fit for the HO model. Optimized parameters can be found in Tab. 2.1.

change of volume has been measured in porcine [64] and canine [65] myocardium to be about 5% under passive biaxial load similar to that at the end of diastole. Likewise, under confined compression changes of up to 10% volumetric strain were observed [64].

Second, when incorporating the material laws into a FEM framework, it is a common approach to loosen the incompressibility constraint a little in exchange for easier computations. These laws are commonly referred to as nearly incompressible and separate additively the total tissue energy density Ψ_{tot} into an isochoric and a volumetric part, thus reading

$$\Psi(\mathbf{F})_{\text{tot}} = \Psi_{\text{iso}}(\bar{\mathbf{F}}) + \Psi_{\text{vol}}(J). \tag{2.26}$$

In order to obtain the isochoric term Ψ_{iso}, one must simply replace all instances of the deformation gradient in the incompressible formulation with its isometric counterpart

$$\mathbf{F} \mapsto \bar{\mathbf{F}} = J^{1/3}\mathbf{F}. \tag{2.27}$$

For the volumetric strain energy density Ψ_{vol}, on the other hand, there is no simple recipe to follow. A plethora of different functions has been proposed over the decades many of which are analyzed in Ref. [66]. Common representatives are

$$\Psi_{\text{vol}}(J) = \begin{cases} \frac{\kappa}{2}(J-1)^2 & [6] \\ \frac{\kappa}{2}(\log J)^2 & [67] \\ \kappa\left(\frac{J^2-1}{2} - \log J\right) & [68] \end{cases} \tag{2.28}$$

the choice among which, in principle, is free as long as the bulk modulus κ is adapted to match the desired (in)compressibility. The example on the bottom of Eq. 2.28 is the one, I employ in this work as it has been used successfully in conjunction with the HO model in the past.

2.3 Finite Element Method

For numerical approximations of differential equations, such as Cauchy's first equation of motion (see Eq. 2.21), there exist several different methods that can be made use of. Popular representatives are the finite difference or finite volume method. However, as it has been developed explicitly with the aim to solve structural mechanics[1] [132] it comes to no surprise that the FEM may pride itself to be the most popular approach in the field. In the following, I sketch the principal ideas of the FEM while for mathematical rigor and elaborate revision of different approaches within the FEM the book of *Hackbusch* [69] is recommended.

Consider a boundary value problem on the domain Ω_0 taking the form

$$\mathcal{L}\mathbf{u} = g(\mathbf{u}) \qquad \text{with} \qquad \mathbf{u} = h(\mathbf{u}) \text{ for } \mathbf{u} \in \partial\Omega_0 \tag{2.29}$$

[1]More precisely: It was researched in a heavy attempt to calculate the stresses arising on the wings of aircrafts.

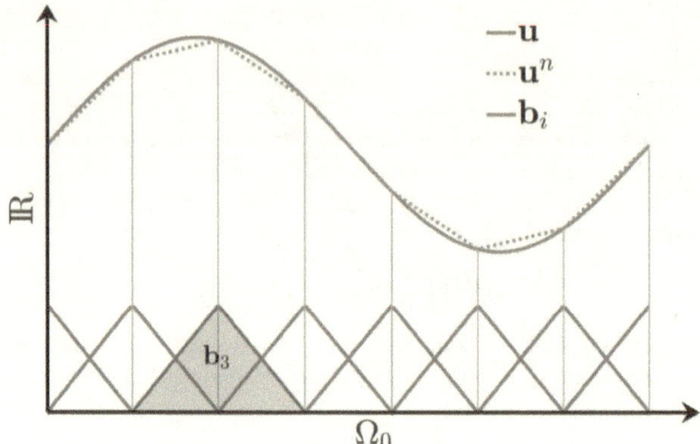

FIGURE 2.4: Schematic for a possible realization of piecewise linear finite elements in a one dimensional domain. The weighted sum of the base functions $\mathbf{b}_i$ approximates the true solution $\mathbf{u}$ (see Ref. [4]).

with differential operator $\mathcal{L}$, inhomogeneity g and boundary values h. Multiplying the differential equation with a test function φ and integrating over the domain Ω_0

$$\int_{\Omega_0} \mathcal{L}(\mathbf{u})\varphi \mathrm{d}V = \int_{\Omega_0} g(\mathbf{u})\varphi \mathrm{d}V \tag{2.30}$$

transforms the *pointwise* formulation into the so-called *weak* formulation by demanding that it must hold regardless of the choice of φ. Contrary to the pointwise formulation, the weak formulation in fact weakens the requirement that Eq. 2.29 should hold on every single point of the domain. Thus, for example, a discontinuity in the first derivative of $\mathbf{u}$ does not object its validity as a solution of the differential equation [4].

Following the *Galerkin* procedure, functions $\mathbf{u}$ and φ are discretized with respect to a linearly independent base system $\{b_1, b_2, \ldots, b_n\}$ with $n \in \mathbb{N}$, the span of which approximates the function space covering all possible solutions, yielding

$$\mathbf{u}^n = \sum_{i=1}^{n} u_i \mathbf{b}_i \qquad \text{and} \qquad \varphi^n = \sum_{i=1}^{n} \phi_i \mathbf{b}_i. \tag{2.31}$$

The functions $\mathbf{b}_i$, $i \in \{1, 2, ..., n\}$ are the eponymous finite elements, a piece wise linear realization of which is depicted in Fig. 2.4. With the definitions

$$\begin{aligned}(\mathbf{L})_{i,j} &= \int_{\Omega_0} \mathbf{b}_i \mathcal{L} \mathbf{b}_j \mathrm{d}V \\ (\mathbf{f})_i &= \int_{\Omega_0} g \mathbf{b}_i \mathrm{d}V\end{aligned} \tag{2.32}$$

finding a solution to the weak formulation of the differential equation can be reduced to solving the linear system of equations

$$\mathbf{L}\mathbf{u}^n = \mathbf{f}. \tag{2.33}$$

Throughout this work, I make use of the software package *COMSOL Multiphysics*™[126] to perform simulations based on the FEM here introduced. As a means to check the validity of the algorithms and their applicability to cardiac deformation simulations, I compared the solutions calculated by *COMSOL* with a set of benchmarks formulated in Ref. [70]. Two of the benchmarks can be found exemplary in Appendix A.

While Fig. 2.4 depicts a set of linear elements, also higher-order polynomials can be consulted, which, if not stated otherwise, are of third-order throughout this work. As the direct solver *PARDISO* is employed, the relative tolerance of which is set to 10^{-3}.

2.4 Klotz Curve

The previous chapters laid out the fundamental formalisms of structural mechanics, which, now, will be put at test by performing a simple experimental analysis. It was found by *Klotz et al.* [71] that the EDPVR can be normalized in such a way that, no matter if dog, rat, or human, all values fall closely onto a single curve, the so-called Klotz curve which can be admired in Fig. 2.5. To match the Klotz curve, the authors made use of a simple exponential ansatz reading

$$p = A_n \bar{V}^{B_n} \ , \quad \text{with} \ \ \bar{V} = \frac{V - V_0}{V_{30} - V_0}. \tag{2.34}$$

The normalized volume $\bar{V}(p)$ comprises volumes measured at different pressure levels p, namely $V_0 = V(0)$ and $V_{30} = V(30\,\mathrm{mmHg})$ The data used for the fitting procedure is provided in Fig. 2.5, yielding the optimal parameters listed in Tab. 2.2.

Eq. 2.34 is an *ad-hoc* function not involving any physical justification. Furthermore, it shows only poor compliance with the experimental data at small volumes. Hence, I propose a novel, yet simplistic, model, based on the exponential energy density provided in Eq. 2.22. Since the EDPVR caters only a single curve, it is an outright overkill to use Eq. 2.22 to its full extend. Instead, only the isotropic term involving the parameters a and b is considered, reading

$$\Psi = \frac{a}{2b}[e^{b(I_1-3)} - 1]. \tag{2.35}$$

With the intention to match this simplicity, also the shape of the heart is reduced to a sphere [72] of inner radius R_{endo} and normalized wall thickness Δ as depicted in Fig. 2.6. Assuming complete incompressibility and purely radial deformation yields the kinematic constraint $\lambda_\theta^2 \lambda_\rho = 1$ with radial and tangential strains λ_ρ and λ_θ respectively. Thus, the first invariant can be expressed as

$$I_1 = \lambda_\rho^2 + 2/\lambda_\rho \tag{2.36}$$

with the radial strain following the expression

$$\lambda_\rho = \frac{R^2}{r^2}, \tag{2.37}$$

with reference and mapped radius R and r respectively. From incompressibility it follows straight forward that

$$R^3 - R_{\text{endo}}^3 = r^3 - r_{\text{endo}}^3 \quad \Rightarrow \quad \hat{r} = \frac{r}{R_{\text{endo}}} = \left(\hat{R}^3 + \hat{V} - 1\right)^{1/3}, \tag{2.38}$$

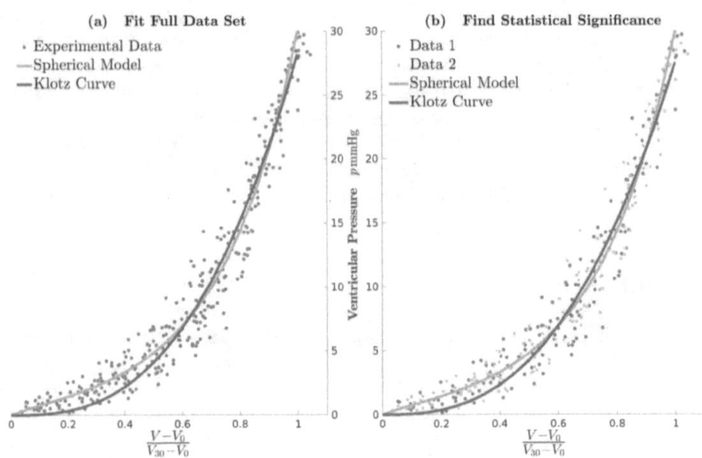

FIGURE 2.5: (a): Comparison of original Klotz-Curve (Eq. 2.34) with the novel, spherical model (Eq. 2.40b). (b) The same functions now fitted to two disjoint subsets of the original data set, namely **Data 1** and **Data 2**. An F-test did not show any significant difference between the two models. All model parameters for (a) and (b) can be found in Tab. 2.2.

where $\hat{R} = R/R_{\text{endo}}$ and $\hat{V} = V/V_0$ are the corresponding normalized reference radius and ventricular volume (VV). The pressure-volume relation for such a setup can be derived in two different ways, both of which are laid out below.

Mechanical Work Approach

Along similar lines as the derivation of Cauchy stress given in Eq. 2.15, let Ω_0 denote the reference geometry of the medium, endowing the total elastic energy

$$W = \int_{\Omega_0} \Psi \mathrm{d}\Omega = \int_{R_{endo}}^{R_{epi}} 4\pi R^2 \Psi(R) \mathrm{d}R. \tag{2.39}$$

From classical mechanics it is known that any mechanical work W performed on the sphere due to a given internal pressure p follows the relation

$$
\begin{aligned}
\mathrm{d}W &= p\mathrm{d}V \\
\Rightarrow p &= 4\pi R_{\text{endo}}^3 \int_{R_{endo}}^{R_{epi}} \hat{R}^2 \frac{\mathrm{d}\Psi}{\mathrm{d}V}\mathrm{d}\hat{R} \\
&= 3V_0 \int_{R_{endo}}^{R_{epi}} \hat{R}^2 \frac{\mathrm{d}\Psi}{\mathrm{d}\lambda_\rho}\frac{\mathrm{d}\lambda_\rho}{\mathrm{d}\hat{V}}\frac{1}{V_0}\mathrm{d}\hat{R} \\
&= \boxed{-2\int_0^{\Delta} \frac{\lambda_\rho^2}{\hat{r}}\frac{\mathrm{d}\Psi}{\mathrm{d}\lambda_\rho}\mathrm{d}\delta} \qquad (2.40\text{a}) \\
&= 2a\int_0^{\Delta} \frac{1-\lambda_\rho^3}{\hat{r}} e^{b(I_1-3)}\mathrm{d}\delta, \qquad (2.40\text{b})
\end{aligned}
$$

where we incorporated the energy density from Eq. 2.35 together with

$$
\frac{\mathrm{d}\lambda_\rho}{\mathrm{d}\hat{V}} = -\frac{2}{3}\frac{\hat{R}^2}{\hat{r}^5}, \qquad (2.41)
$$

which follows directly from substituting Eq. 2.38 into Eq. 2.37.

Stress Approach

While the work approach appeals to the heart of physicists, the following is more popular among engineers, especially those working with any kind of pressure vessel. Taking the cross-section of the sphere, I find that the change in total radial force must be balanced by the total stress along the circumference of the cross-section, leading to the force balance

$$
\begin{aligned}
\partial_r \pi r^2 \sigma_\rho &= 2\pi r \sigma_\theta \\
\Rightarrow 2r\sigma_\rho + r^2\partial_r\sigma_\rho &= 2r\sigma_\theta \\
\Rightarrow \sigma_\rho(r_{\text{endo}}) = p &= \boxed{2\int_{r_{endo}}^{r_{epi}} \frac{\sigma_\theta - \sigma_\rho}{r}\mathrm{d}r} \qquad (2.42)
\end{aligned}
$$

with the boundary conditions $\sigma_\rho(r_{\text{epi}}) = 0$ and $\sigma_\rho(r_{\text{endo}}) = p$. Considering the equalities

$$
\begin{aligned}
\sigma_\rho &= \lambda_\rho\partial_{\lambda_\rho}\Psi - \tilde{p}\,, & \sigma_\theta &= \lambda_\theta\partial_{\lambda_\theta}\Psi - \tilde{p}, \\
\lambda_\rho\mathrm{d}\delta &= \mathrm{d}r, \quad \text{and} & \frac{\mathrm{d}}{\mathrm{d}\lambda_\rho} &= \partial_{\lambda_\rho} + 2(\partial_{\lambda_\rho}\lambda_\theta)\partial_{\lambda_\theta}, \qquad (2.43)
\end{aligned}
$$

where $\tilde{p}$ depicts the hydrostatic pressure responsible for the incompressible deformation, one can easily convert Eq. 2.42 into Eq. 2.40a. For very thin pressure vessels $\Delta \ll 1$ Eq. 2.42 simplifies to the well known Laplace's law [133]

$$
\sigma = \frac{p\hat{r}}{2\Delta}, \qquad (2.44)
$$

where σ is the membrane stress disregarding hydrostatic pressure.

A consistency check presented in Fig. 2.6 shows how well theory and simulation align. Fitting Eq. 2.40b to the Klotz-Data yields the parameters presented in Tab. 2.2.

While the parameter a describes the Young's modulus of the material at low stretches, b represents nonlinear stiffening. The third parameter Δ characterizes an interspecies average of the relative thickness of the left ventricle and is in good agreement with the value for human wall thickness as calculated in Eq. 4.25.

With the aim to quantify whether the power law or the spherical model is better suited as a fit function, I perform an F-test, which necessitates independent data points for the two models to be compared. Thus, I randomly divide the original dataset from Fig. 2.5(a) into the two subsets shown in Fig. 2.5(b), which, then, are used for the two independent fits. For a single realization of this scheme, the Fisher function

$$F = \frac{\chi_1^2/f_1}{\chi_2^2/f_2} \tag{2.45}$$

is used, where index 1 represents the spherical model, while 2 refers to the power law, and f_i is the respective amount of degrees of freedom. The result obtained is $F_\rho = 1.1$. For a Fischer-statistic, the probability to find values more extreme than this result is $P(F > F_\rho) = 26\%$ thus making the outcome all but significant. On the contrary, for these subsets, χ^2 takes values favoring in fact the power law whereas the full set favors the spherical model. From a statistical point of view, henceforth, there is no preference for either of the two models.

However, the spherical model shows clear strengths for small volumes as it shows a positive linear slope there. It is also worth mentioning that, contrary to this model, the power law is not constrained to match p(1)=30 mmHg. This opens a new degree of freedom, which naturally promotes smaller errors. Nonetheless, violating this constraint is an actual flaw for computer simulations, since there, by design, it is always met. The Klotz curve is widely used as a reference value in *in vivo* parameter estimation using computational simulations [60, 73, 74]. In the largest part, such simulations incorporate exponential energy densities and thus show stronger similarity to Eq. 2.40b. Hence, in such studies, I recommend the use of the idealized sphere over the power law for better comparability.

	Spherical Model, Eq. 2.40b				Power Law, Eq. 2.34		
	Δ	a [kPa]	b	χ^2	A_n [kPa]	B_n	χ^2
Full Data	0.27 ±0.29	1.15±0.7	3.8± 0.5	1007	3.7	2.76	1060
Subset	0.27± 0.42	1.1±1	3.83±0.71	530	3.672±0.048	2.697±0.071	483

TABLE 2.2: Least square fits for the two different models with respect to the data presented in Fig. 2.5. Please note, that this solution is not unique as the creation of subsets involves randomization. Although the error estimates are rather large for the spherical model, especially with regards to Δ, the result for the random subsample shows remarkable similarity to the full data set, thus reinforcing the trust in their precision.

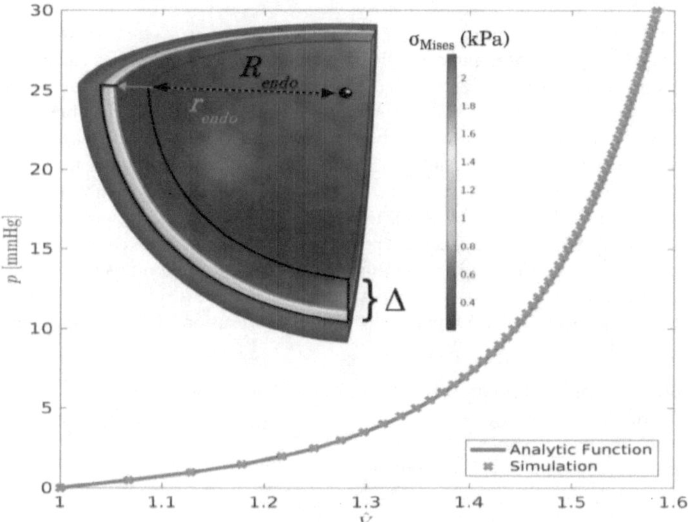

FIGURE 2.6: The simulation for $1/8^{th}$ of a sphere with symmetry BCs shows great accordance to the analytical expression. The von Mises stress (Ref. [49] Eq. 2) is colorcoded. These results were created with the parameters $\Delta = 0.23, a = 1.6576\,\text{kPa}$ and $b = 13.9218$. Note that Δ resembles the normalized thickness of the ventricle in the reference configuration.

Chapter 3

Fibre Dispersion

3.1 A Little Tribute to Fiber Reinforced Materials

As laid out in Sec. 1.1.1 fibers play a crucial role in the mechanics of myocardium. The collagen lends its robustness to withstand stretch under diastolic inflation while the cardiomyocytes display their strength when contracting during systole. A fibrous structure also plays a crucial role for example in arteries, where the fiber angle determines its resistance to pressure load as shown in Fig. 3.2c. The versatility of fiber reinforced materials, however, goes far beyond muscle, collagen or even animal tissue. Bamboo, for instance, just like other grasses, inherits its bending flexibility from tiny vessels as shown in Fig. 3.2b allowing it to grow sightly 25 m tall while preserving a slim waist of mere 20 cm in diameter, thus making it a formidable construction material. Similarly, engineering makes great use of fiber reinforced composites like concrete or laminates to fabricate materials with anisotropic mechanical properties. Whenever a new material, just like EHM, is designed, the distribution of the comprising fibers is of prime importance.

Henceforth, it comes to no surprise that the fiber architecture of myocardium has been researched extensively since the late 1960s[1] [57, 75–79], the results of which are discussed in detail in Sec. 4.3.1. Also the influence of changes of the mean fiber orientation on cardiac performance has been studied *in silico* recently [80]. However, to the best of my knowledge, there is no study that tests experimentally the robustness of constitutive laws with respect to mean fiber orientation. It is unclear, whether a HO model, which has been fitted to experimental shear experiments as shown in Fig. 2.3, still can describe the same tissue specimen if the fiber orientation has slightly changed (which is equivalent to performing the same simple shear experiment with a slightly tilted cut plane). In Fig. 3.1 the predictions of the HO model with respect to such a change are demonstrated.

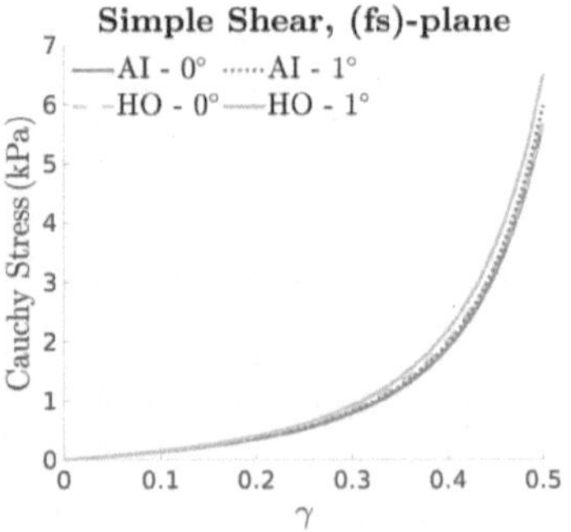

FIGURE 3.1: Variation under in-plane fiber rotation of 1° for a dispersion afflicted (angular integration (AI), see Ref. [49]) and a dispersion free (HO) model. Both models were matched to the same experimental data with zero fiber rotation, displayed in Fig. 2.3. Predicted stresses are elevated for the HO model, exhibiting a 15% increase through rotation *vs.* a 5% increase for the AI model.

[1] In fact, first documentations reach much further into the past. Already Leonardo da Vinci mapped the helical fiber orientation of the heart [81].

It is quite surprising that a reorientation of a mere degree, which is hardly detectable in advance of the actual simple shear experiment, yields already deviations from the original value by 15%. As we show in Sec. 3.2, this strong directional sensitivity can be reduced after inclusion of a new ingredient - **Dispersion**.

The HO model treats myocardium to be comprised of unidirectional fibers, but

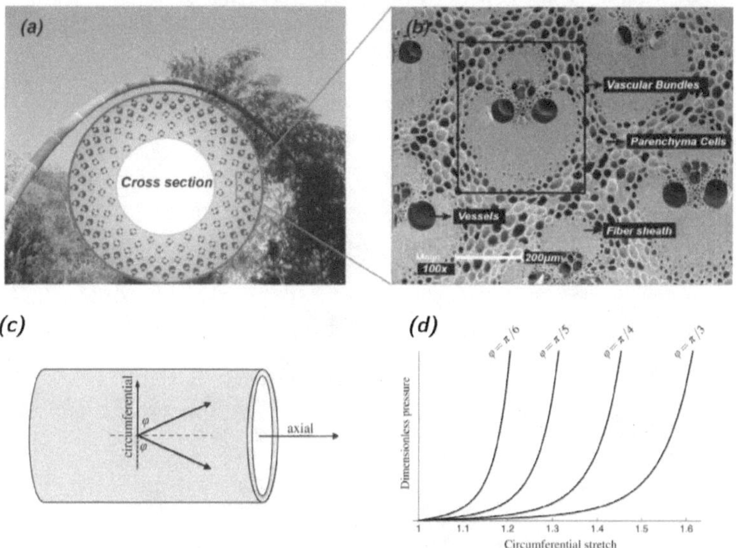

FIGURE 3.2: (a): Schematic cross section through a moso bamboo revealing the fiber pores which are responsible for the bending flexibility (taken from Ref. [82] with permission). (b) Field emission scanning electron microscope micrograph of the structure of bamboo with its different constituents. (c) Artery schematic depicting the opening angle ϕ between two collagen fiber families which influences the resistance to blood pressure (d). The better the fibers align with the circumferential direction the less the artery stretches under increased blood pressure. Fig. (c) and (d) are taken from Ref. [19] with permission.

nature is not this precise. Instead, fibers are randomly distributed about their mean direction. This randomization smooths the impact of small alterations in the mean fiber orientation as demonstrated in Fig. 3.1, thus easing computational simulations that otherwise would get stuck in numerical instabilities. Interestingly, small dispersion coefficients[2] already yield a strong impact on model predictions. More importantly, also the choice of dispersion model highly impacts the prediction for a change in fiber orientation. This opens a huge ambiguity, which models are actually valid for a given problem and it mandates new experimental tests to rule out the right one.

In the following paper [49], we present a novel class of dispersion models, which, among other features, compute faster and are easier to implement into a numeric

[2]The smaller the dispersion coefficient the narrower the fiber dispersion distribution given by Eq. 4 Ref. [49].

scheme than comparable predecessors and although, originally, they have been tailored to serve for cardiac mechanics simulation, these models can be applied to any soft material undergoing large deformations and which comprises individual fibers displaying an exponential strain energy. I contributed in large extents to this publication as I formulated the principle idea and performed all corresponding calculations either by hand or with the aid of *Mathematica* [127], the basic functions of which can be found in Appendix C. In addition, I prepared all simulations as well as the postprocessing and wrote large proportions of the text.

PHYSICAL REVIEW APPLIED **13,** 064039 (2020)

Structure Tensors for Dispersed Fibers in Soft Materials

Moritz Kalhöfer-Köchling,[1,2] Eberhard Bodenschatz,[1,2,3,4] and Yong Wang[1,2,3,*]

[1] *Max Planck Institute for Dynamics and Self-Organization, 37077 Göttingen, Germany*
[2] *German Center for Cardiovascular Research, Partner Site Göttingen, 37075 Göttingen, Germany*
[3] *Institute for Dynamics of Complex Systems, University of Göttingen, 37073 Göttingen, Germany*
[4] *Laboratory of Atomic and Solid-State Physics and Sibley School of Mechanical and Aerospace Engineering, Cornell University, Ithaca, New York 14853, USA*

(Received 3 February 2020; revised manuscript received 4 May 2020; accepted 19 May 2020; published 16 June 2020)

Soft tissues, such as skin, myocardium, and chordae tendineae, typically display anisotropic mechanical behavior due to their fibrous nature. In constitutive modeling, fiber families frequently are assumed to be unidirectional. Recent numerical results, however, display the need to incorporate dispersion of fiber orientation. This evidence gets supplemented by new experimental results based on high-resolution second-harmonic imaging microscopy. Generalized structure-tensor (GST) models are frequently utilized to model fiber dispersion, as they are mathematically easy to treat and demand only a little effort to implement. They can be regarded as Taylor-series expansions of the numerically more challenging angular-integration (AI) method, which encompasses a distribution of fiber orientations together with the associated fiber stress. In this work, we show how low-order GST models give rise to numerical instabilities as they show strong sensitivity with regards to the mean fiber orientation. To overcome these instabilities, we propose a different class of GST models, termed squared GST (SGST), which computes faster, is easier to implement, and converges to the AI faster than previous GST models of similar order. The SGST models promise to be adaptable to generalized problems, such as functional decomposition of fiber density as well as coupling between different fiber families. Advanced simulations with the proposed models will shed light on the complex behavior of fiber reinforced soft materials.

DOI: 10.1103/PhysRevApplied.13.064039

I. INTRODUCTION

Whether it is neurons, myocytes, or collagen, most soft biological tissues comprise fibers leading to anisotropic mechanical behavior [1,2]. In disease, alteration of mechanical properties of tissues is a valuable biomarker for diagnosis. Since material stiffness is not always accessible directly via state-of-the-art medical measurements, computer simulations are becoming a critical tool in both disease diagnosis and treatment [3–5], necessitating robust numerical and mathematical models to characterize architecture and orientation of fibers.

Evidenced by recent findings [6,7], unidirectional fiber models are insufficient to describe tissue mechanics and thus dispersion of fiber orientation should be included. Concerning constitutive modeling, there are two schools debating how to treat fiber dispersion mathematically. The first is dating back to Lanir [8], who proposes to attribute an elastic energy to every single fiber, the orientation of which follows a given angular distribution. Then, angular integration (AI) of said energy gives rise to the macroscopic response to external loading. The second school, on the other hand, follows the steps of Gasser *et al.* [6], who translate the fiber architecture into a generalized structure tensor (GST), which describes collective fiber deformation. Both schools, expectedly, carry their own advantages and disadvantages. The AI furnishes a bottom up, easy to understand energy density while on the other hand, in finite-element simulation, it involves the task of integrating over angle space on each iteration for every single Gauss point, which quickly becomes heavily time consuming. The GST models, in contrast, are easy to implement and fast to simulate since many calculations can be precomputed. In return, exclusion of fibers under compression is difficult [9] but necessary to account for the fact that they usually buckle under compressive loads.

As GST models can be interpreted as low-order Taylor-series expansions of the AI model, the former have been criticized for their lack of accuracy as stated by

*yong.wang@ds.mpg.de

Refs. [10–12]. Conversely, it has been shown by Holzapfel *et al.* [13] that both models approximate experimental data equally well.

Although both, the GST and the AI, models can be matched to the same experiment, they show large differences in their predictions if small changes in the fiber architecture are introduced. Especially for simple shear the sensitivity to the fiber arrangement is substantial, which is highlighted in Fig. 1. Directional sensitivity, shown in Fig. 1(b), measures how much shear stresses change relatively if the mean fiber orientation is altered. Taking, for example, the (fn_1) shear mode with a shear of $\gamma = 0.2$, a dispersionless (HO) and a classical GST model (0GST) deviate in stress by roughly 25% if the fibers are rotated by only 1°, contrary to the AI model, which varies only by roughly 5%. This behavior becomes even more pronounced for smaller shear values or the $(n_1 f)$ shear mode.

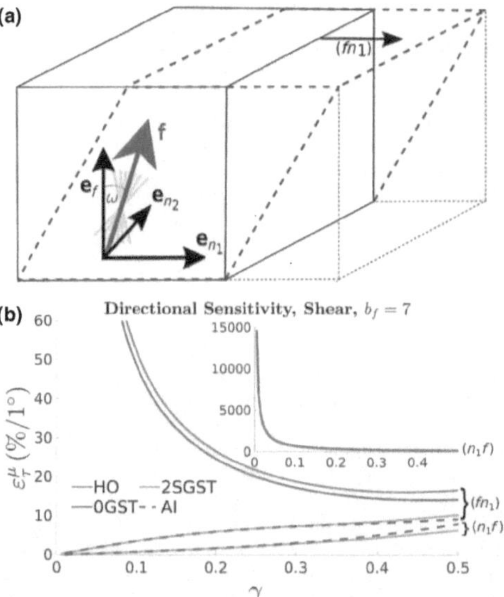

FIG. 1. Directional sensitivity for simple shear. (a) Geometric setup for simple shear with the frame showing original mean fiber orientation ($\mathbf{e}_f$) and two normal directions ($\mathbf{e}_{n_1}, \mathbf{e}_{n_2}$). Unit vector **f** portrays the mean fiber direction after rotation ω in the (fn_1) plane. Solid lines depict the reference configuration versus the deformed one represented by dashed lines. Dotted lines visualize the shear γ. In (b) the resulting relative change shear stress ε_τ^μ as defined in Eq. (18) shows that directional sensitivity depends heavily on the degree to which dispersion is embedded in the model (HO > 0GST > 2GST > AI, cf. Sec. V). All models incorporate the same elastic parameter $b_f = 7$ and $a_f = 1$. Shear mode $(n_1 f)$ for the 0GST model is shown as an inset while the corresponding value for the HO model diverges.

As we show in this work, directional sensitivity plays a key role in numerical stability even if only small shear deformations are present. While for most ordinary shapes, said sensitivity is negligible, it becomes essential, once realistic conditions with irregular shapes, such as cardiac infarctions or wounds, are considered. To prevent instabilities arising from sensitivities, we develop a class of GST models, termed squared generalized structure-tensor (SGST) models, which closely match the directional sensitivity of the AI model [cf. 2SGST in Fig. 1(b)], while still offering the framework of classical GST models, yielding an easy implementation and rapid numerical calculation. The approach entails the Taylor-series expansion, which shows faster convergence to the AI, and is mathematically easier to implement for higher-order terms, while, at the same time, reducing computational costs compared to conventional GST models of the same order.

The general framework incorporates an exponential fiber strain energy, which has proven successful to describe cardiac [14–16] as well as aortic [6,17,18] tissue in experiment and simulation likewise. The dispersion of fiber angles is governed by the von Mises distribution, which is supported by recent experiments on human myocardium [19] and aortic tissue [20], although our approach can be applied to more general fiber arrangements.

An easy-to-use MATLAB library, comprising the different models up to sixth polynomial order, is provided as Supplemental Material [21].

II. CONSTITUTIVE MODELING OF DISPEPRSED FIBERS

Following a commonly used macroscopic framework, we assume that deformation is governed by an affine map $\mathbf{x} = \chi(\mathbf{X})$, which smoothly transforms a material point $\mathbf{X}$ in the stress-free state into the spatial frame $\mathbf{x}$. The deformation gradient, then, is defined as $\mathbf{F} = \partial\mathbf{x}/\partial\mathbf{X}$, with the determinant $J = \det(\mathbf{F})$ measuring local volume changes (incompressibility corresponds to $J \equiv 1$). Multiplicative decomposition $\mathbf{F} = (J^{1/3}\mathbb{I})\overline{\mathbf{F}}$ splits the deformation gradient into a distortional $\overline{\mathbf{F}}$ and a dilational part $J^{1/3}\mathbb{I}$. Postulating perfect bonding between ground matrix and fibers, we ignore microscopic nonaffine deformations [22]. The strain of an individual fiber $\mathbf{f}'$, thus, follows the simple relation $\epsilon^2 = \overline{\mathbf{E}} : \mathbf{M}$, with isochoric Green-Lagrange strain $\overline{\mathbf{E}}$ and structure tensor $\mathbf{M}$ defined as

$$\overline{\mathbf{E}} = \frac{1}{2}(\overline{\mathbf{F}}^{\mathrm{T}}\overline{\mathbf{F}} - \mathbb{I}), \quad \mathbf{M} = \mathbf{f}' \otimes \mathbf{f}', \tag{1}$$

where $\mathbb{I}$ is the identity tensor. The AI for an arbitrary function g is defined as the average $\langle\cdot\rangle$ over the solid angle [8]

$$\langle g\rangle = \frac{N_{\text{fiber}}}{4\pi}\int_0^{\pi}\int_0^{2\pi}\rho[\mathbf{f}'(\Theta,\phi)]g(\Theta,\phi)\sin\Theta d\phi d\Theta, \tag{2}$$

where the fiber density per volume $N_{\text{fiber}} = 1$ w.l.o.g. and $\rho[\mathbf{f}'(\Theta,\phi)]$ is the fiber density per solid angle $d\Omega = \sin\theta d\phi d\theta$. Assuming an energy density $\psi_f(\epsilon)$ of an individual fiber, the AI yields the total fiber energy density

$$\Psi_f = \langle\psi_f(\epsilon)\rangle. \tag{3}$$

As it has been used successfully to describe, for example, mammalian myocardium (human [19] and dog [23]) as well as arterial walls [6], we focus our attention on the von Mises distribution

$$\rho(\Theta) = 4\sqrt{\frac{b_\rho}{2\pi}}\frac{\exp(b_\rho[\cos(2\Theta)+1])}{\operatorname{erfi}(\sqrt{2b_\rho})}, \tag{4}$$

which is controlled through dispersion coefficient b_ρ. It is centered about $\Theta = 0$ representing the mean fiber orientation $\mathbf{e}_f$ and shows rotational symmetry. The latter attribute is chosen for convenience, although the following analysis can be applied to more general, asymmetric distributions. For biological fibers, exponential stiffening is most commonly observed and can be expressed using [17]

$$\psi_f(\epsilon) = \frac{a_f}{2b_f}\left(e^{4b_f\epsilon^4} - 1\right), \tag{5}$$

where a_f and b_f comprise linear and nonlinear elastic material properties. Using finite-element methods (FEM) to simulate such material requires repetitive numerical calculation of Eq. (2) on each time step for every single Gauss point, thus making it heavily time consuming. Contrary to the exponential energy function shown in Eq. (5), trigonometric functions can easily be integrated, inspiring the use of GST. Classically, the GST $\mathbf{H}$ is defined as [6]

$$\mathbf{H} = \langle\mathbf{M}\rangle = \kappa\mathbb{I} + (1-3\kappa)\mathbf{M}(\Theta = 0, \phi = 0), \tag{6}$$

together with structure parameter κ

$$\kappa = \frac{1}{2}\langle\sin^2(\theta)\rangle, \tag{7}$$

which, in three dimensions, is confined to the interval $[0, 1/3]$, where 0 reflects unidirectional behavior while 1/3 embodies complete isotropy. Following an approach similar to Ref. [11], $\mathbf{H}$ can be used as an anchor point for

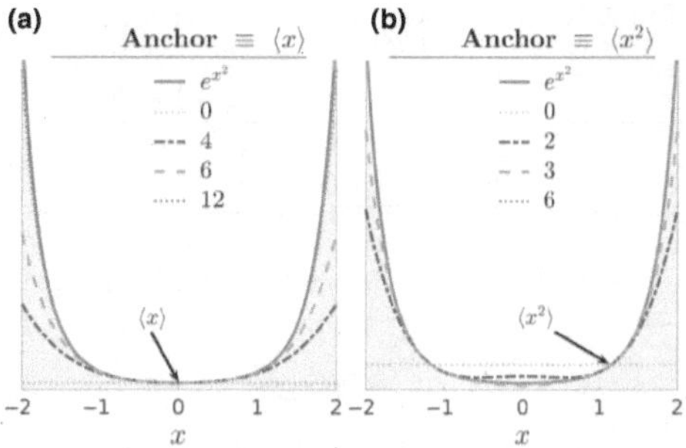

FIG. 2. Taylor series of $f(x) = e^{x^2}$ performed for two different anchor points. The numerals in the respective legends signify the order to which the Taylor series is performed. If this number, in the case of (b), is multiplied by 2 the product matches the polynomial order in x of (a). The area shaded in light blue signifies the integral to be approximated.

a Taylor-series expansion of Eq. (2). Using multi-index notation, the nth-order approximation is defined as

$$\Psi_f^{n\text{GST}} = \sum_{|\alpha|\le n}\frac{D^\alpha\psi_f(\langle\epsilon^2\rangle)}{\alpha!}\langle(\mathbf{M}-\mathbf{H})^\alpha\rangle. \tag{8}$$

The zeroth-order term, consequently, reads

$$\Psi_f^{0\text{GST}} = \frac{a_f}{2b_f}e^{4b_f(\mathbf{E}:\mathbf{H})^2} = \psi_f(\langle\epsilon^2\rangle^2). \tag{9}$$

Using Jensen's inequality, however, we find that

$$\langle\psi_f(\epsilon^4)\rangle \ge \psi_f(\langle\epsilon^4\rangle) \ge \psi_f(\langle\epsilon^2\rangle^2), \tag{10}$$

which sparks the idea that $\langle\epsilon^4\rangle$ promises to be better suited as an anchor point for the Taylor expansion, as we later confirm in Sec. III. The effects of this paradigm shift are showcased in Fig. 2, where the averages of two different Taylor series of the function f

$$\langle f(x)\rangle = \langle e^{x^2}\rangle = \frac{\sqrt{\pi}}{4}\operatorname{erfi}(2) \tag{11}$$

are compared. For demonstration purposes, here, we focus on the simple case of a one-dimensional function and the average $\langle\cdot\rangle$ performed with respect to a homogeneous probability density on the interval $[-2, 2]$. It is evident that anchor point $\langle x^2\rangle$ shows faster convergence, and closer proximity to Eq. (11), which is highlighted for small orders in x in Table I.

TABLE I. Taylor series of Eq. (11) for two different anchor points ($\langle x\rangle$ and $\langle x^2\rangle$) and different polynomial orders n_x.

n_x	0	2	4	6	8	10	12	∞
$\langle x\rangle$	1	$2.\overline{3}$	$3.9\overline{3}$	5.46	6.64	7.42	7.86	8.23
$\langle x^2\rangle$	3.79	3.79	6.491	7.18	7.86	8.08	8.18	

We, therefore, define the squared generalized structure tensor

$$\mathbf{H_2} = \langle \mathbf{M} \otimes \mathbf{M} \rangle, \tag{12}$$

which yields a corresponding class of fiber-dispersion models

$$\Psi_f^{n\mathrm{SGST}} = \sum_{|\alpha|\leq n} \frac{D^\alpha \psi_f(\langle \epsilon^4 \rangle)}{\alpha!} \langle (\mathbf{M}\otimes\mathbf{M} - \mathbf{H_2})^\alpha \rangle, \tag{13}$$

which computes faster, approximates the AI model more closely, and is mathematically easier to handle than GST models of identical order in ϵ^2. All structure tensors needed for a Taylor expansion up to second order can be found in the Appendix together with Eq. (6).

III. PROXIMITY ANALYSIS

In the following, we quantify the relation between AI, GST, and SGST models analytically through variations in stresses. Therefore, we adopt fiber stress $\overline{\sigma}^\mu$ for an incompressible material [16]

$$\overline{\sigma}^\mu = \mathbf{F} \frac{\partial \Psi_f^\mu}{\partial \mathbf{E}} \mathbf{F}^T - p(J)\mathbb{I}, \tag{14}$$

where $\mu \in \{\text{2GST,4GST,0SGST,2SGST}\}$ specifies the model of interest, and $p(J)$ is the Lagrangian multiplyer function conserving incompressibility. We confine our analysis to the loading protocol $\mathbb{T}$ comprising biaxial stretch and simple shear. As depicted in Fig. 1, model predictions heavily rely on fiber architecture, wherefore $\mathbb{T}$ includes fibers rotated in (fn_1) plane by angle ω. Together with the different biaxial stretch ratios β we consider the following loading protocols:

$$\begin{aligned}\mathbb{T}_{\text{shear}} &= [(fn_1, \omega), (n_1 f, \omega), (n_1 n_2, \omega) | \omega \in (0^\circ, 45^\circ)],\\ \mathbb{T}_{\text{biax}} &= \Big\{ (ff, \omega, \beta), (n_1 n_1, \omega, \beta) | \omega \in (0^\circ, 45^\circ)\\ &\quad \wedge \beta \in \Big[\Big(1:\frac{1}{2}\Big), \Big(1:\frac{3}{4}\Big), (1:1),\\ &\quad \Big(1:\frac{4}{3}\Big), (1:2)\Big]\Big\}.\end{aligned} \tag{15}$$

The choice for the exponent b_f, which defines the nonlinear elastic fiber response, is loosely based on a parameter estimation attributed to the AI for experimental data for human hearts acquired by Sommer *et al.* [15,19].

As a metric of accuracy for a single realization of fiber distribution belonging to dispersion coefficient $\kappa \sim b_\rho$ [see Eq. (7)], we define the local relative error (LRE)

$$\Delta_\kappa^{\text{LRE},\mu}(\mathbb{T}, \gamma) = \sqrt{\sum_{t\in\mathbb{T}} \left(1 - \frac{\sigma_t^\mu(\gamma)}{\sigma_t^{\text{AI}}(\gamma)}\right)^2 \Big/ ||\mathbb{T}||}, \tag{16}$$

where γ describes the current shear or stretch depending on the loading protocol, and the normalization coefficient $||\mathbb{T}||$ denotes the cardinality of the set of experiments. Models corresponding to first-order terms are not listed since they are equivalent to the zeroth-order terms. Building on the local error estimate, we also define an accumulated or averaged error. It serves as an estimate for the accountability of a given model for a specific choice of κ. As such, we define the averaged relative error (ARE)

$$\Delta^{\text{ARE},\mu}(\mathbb{T}, \kappa) = \sqrt{\int_{\gamma_{\min}}^{\gamma_{\max}} \frac{\Delta_\kappa^{\text{LRE},\mu}(\mathbb{T}, \gamma)^2}{\gamma_{\max} - \gamma_{\min}} d\gamma}, \tag{17}$$

with $(\gamma_{\min}, \gamma_{\max}) = (0, 0.5)$ for simple shear and $(\gamma_{\min}, \gamma_{\max}) = (1, 1.1)$ for biaxial stretch.

The resultant proximity estimates are displayed in Fig. 3. Therein, plots (a) and (d) display how accurately the different models match the AI for a dispersion coefficient $\kappa = 0.06$, which is taken from Ref. [19]. The corresponding LRE plotted in the second column for the same choice of parameters as in the first column, are consulted for better comparability. The double logarithmic plot of the LRE shows nicely how different orders of approximation scale linearly with the deformation coefficient γ. It becomes apparent that the accuracy of the 2GST is related to 0SGST while 4GST is related to 2SGST in their approximation behavior. In the case of $\kappa = 0.06$ we calculate the AI model with numerical schemes offered by *Mathematica*, where we chose an accuracy of 16 digits. As this numerical accuracy is exhausted, further numerical errors impact the LRE, which explains the little kinks in Fig. 3(b), which emerge as $\varepsilon_\tau^{\text{2SGST/4GST}} \to 10^{-7}$.

It has to be remarked, that for biaxial tests, the 4GST model shows much larger relative errors than the 2SGST. Eventually, these errors even exceed those of the 0SGST and 2GST models as γ increases, which is a natural result of the different scaling. As large stretch values dominate the ARE, we can observe corresponding peaks at approximately $\kappa = 0.1$ in Figs. 3(c) and 3(f), heavily suggesting not to use the 4GST model for the chosen range of deformation γ. Conversely, we find that in all categories, the 2SGST model shows lowest errors within the

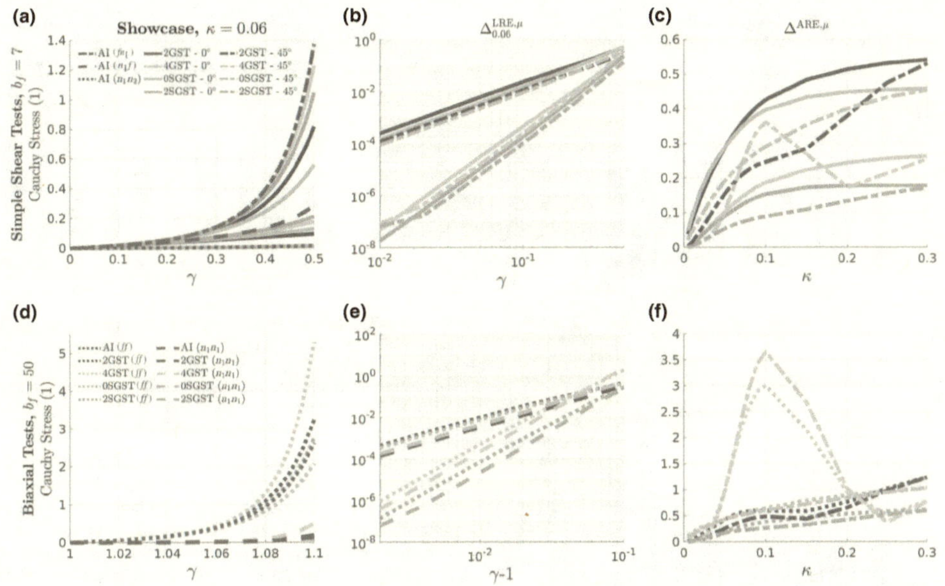

FIG. 3. (a)–(c) Proximity analysis for the two different model classes nGST [Eq. (8)] and nSGST [Eq. (13)] to the AI [Eq. (2)] in the case of simple shear with $a_f = 1$ and $b_f = 7$. They share a common legend from (a). (d)–(f) The same analysis for biaxial stretch, where $b_f = 50$. They share a common legend from (d). (a),(d) Representative Cauchy stress for simple shear and equibiaxial stretch, respectively, with $\kappa = 0.06$, which can be interpreted as 20% isotropy. (b),(e) Local relative errors $\Delta_\kappa^{\mathrm{LRE},\mu}$ [Eq. (16)] with all parameters chosen as in (a),(d). The logarithmic scale reveals at which power in shear or strain the AI is approximated. (c),(f) are concerned with the accumulated relative error $\Delta^{\mathrm{ARE},\mu}$ [Eq. (17)] for different degrees of dispersion, ranging from unidirectional ($\kappa = 0$) to complete isotropic ($\kappa = 1/3$) behavior. Since the (n_1n_2) mode for shear and the (n_1n_1) mode for biaxial stretch yield relatively small stresses, the different models overlap in plots (a),(c).

boundaries considered, making it a promising candidate for simulation.

With a fixed dispersion coefficient κ we can analyze how the ARE changes as the polynomial order n gets further increased. Figure 4 confirms the counterintuitive increase of the $\Delta^{\mathrm{ARE},n\mathrm{GST}}$ with $\kappa = 0.06$ as discussed above. For biaxial tests and simple shear tests incorporating fibers rotated by 45° in the (fn_1) plane this tendency even proceeds beyond $n = 10$, thus discouraging the use of nGST models as an approximation to the AI. For the corresponding $n/2$SGST models depicted, on the other hand, the ARE shows a desired decreasing tendency. Of course this picture is by no means complete and different loading protocols can lead to strikingly divergent error estimates, both for the GST and SGST model classes. Hence, a careful consideration of the occurring loading protocols together with the desired accuracy should shed light on the viability of a given approximation scheme before simulation.

IV. NUMERICAL EFFICIENCY

Quantifying numerical efficency is important to evaluate advantages and disadvantages of an approximation scheme. Nonetheless, finding an appropriate metric for the numerical efficiency of the AI model is difficult as it depends not only on the quadrature rule, and precision requirements used, but it is also heavily influenced by the deformation gradient **F** as well as the dispersion coefficient b_ρ. For best comparability with the results presented in Secs. III and V, we constrain our analysis to simple shear and equibiaxial tests, examining the same range of shear and extension values γ as there.

In order to keep the efficiency estimation independent of any additional algorithms used in a FEM solver, we restrain it to algebraic computation times of the individual AI, SGST, and GST expressions. The resulting computation times can be found in Fig. 5. All calculations are performed with *Mathematica* on a Windows 10

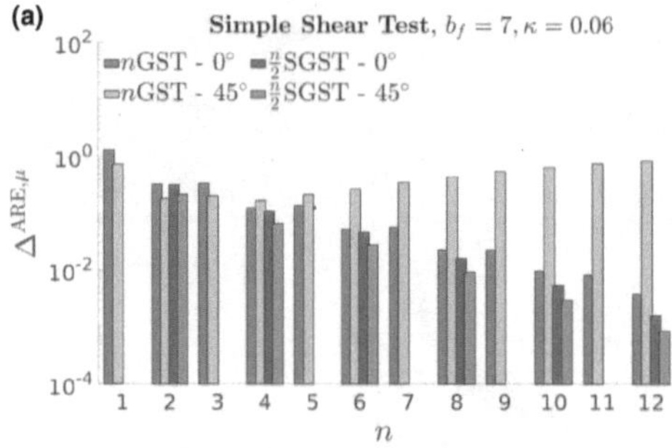

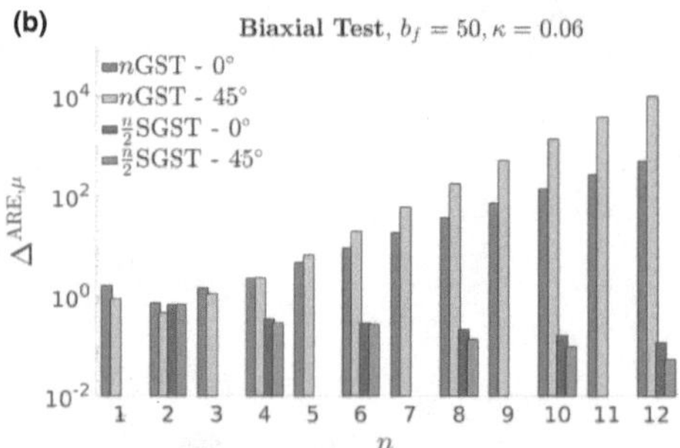

FIG. 4. Averaged relative error as defined in Eq. (17) for different polynomial orders n similar as in Figs. 3(c) and 3(e) with constant dispersion coefficient κ. Clearly, an increase of n does not imply smaller errors for the GST model, contrasting the continuous decline for the SGST model.

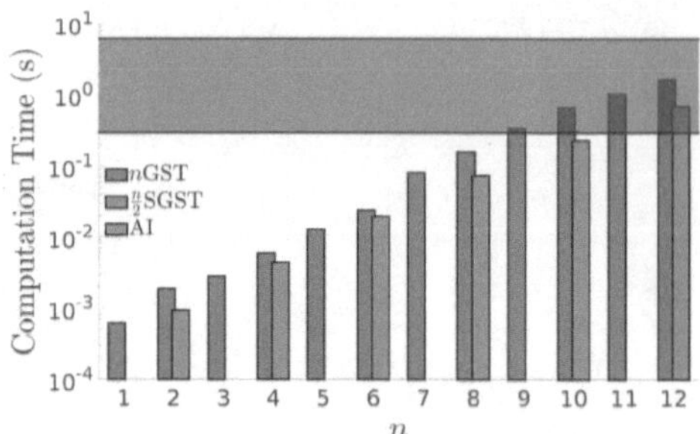

FIG. 5. Algebraic computation times for individual realizations of the GST and SGST model classes, grouped with regards to similar error scaling as presented in Figs. 3(b) and 3(e). The purple region represents the domain of observed computation times for the AI with a precision of eight digits.

computer with an Intel® Core™ i5-7400 CPU and 8GB of memory. For the AI model we utilize an inbuilt global adaptive quadrature rule employing a working precision of eight decimals.

As shown in Fig. 5 the computation time increases exponentially with the order to which the Taylor series is performed. For identical values of $n \in \{2, 4, \ldots, 12\}$, the nGST model takes about 25–180% more time compared with the $n/2$SGST model. This result gets supplemented by calculations performed with our MATLAB library [21], where 4GST takes roughly 25% more computing time compared with its counterpart 2SGST. Such a trend can be attributed to the overall larger algebraic complexity of nGST polynomials. Beyond an order of $n = 10$ the prevalence of the $n/2$SGST model class over the AI becomes questionable, as shown in Fig. 5.

V. DIRECTIONAL SENSITIVITY

When measuring the mean fiber orientation of a given specimen experimentally, such a task can be very difficult, not only because fibers in reality can show strong dispersion, but also because for most tissues this mean fiber orientation is not constant on scales, which stress measurements are performed on. If the model used shows strong dependence on the actual fiber orientation, systematic measurement errors are amplified. As a result, when choosing a model to match experimental results, not only good statistical agreement, but also small systematic errors should be accounted for.

In the case of simple shear, fibers initially are aligned with the cube's perimeters as graphed in Fig. 1(a). As before, let ω denote the angle between the assumed and the true mean fiber orientation in the (fn_1) plane, then, the relative change in predicted stress for a given model μ is computed via

$$\varepsilon_\tau^\mu = \frac{1}{\overline{\sigma}_\tau^\mu} \frac{\partial \overline{\sigma}_\tau^\mu}{\partial \omega}, \tag{18}$$

where $\tau \in \mathbb{T}$. When there is no dispersion ($\mu = \text{HO}$, as proposed by Holzapfel and Ogden [16]), i.e., when $\kappa = 0$, Eq. (18) can be calculated analytically

$$\varepsilon_\tau^{\text{HO}}(\gamma) = \begin{cases} \dfrac{3 + 4b_f \gamma^4}{\gamma} & \tau = (fn_1) \\ \infty & \tau \in \{(n_1 f), (n_1 n_2)\} \\ 0 & \text{else} \end{cases} \tag{19}$$

in the case of simple shear. Figure 1(b) shows how directional sensitivity $\varepsilon_\tau^{\text{HO}}$ diverges for several different loads, which can lead to undetermined fiber orientations in simulation.

Clearly, dispersion decreases this sensitivity, since such an arrangement supports loads of different directions. Consequently, studies investigating the dependency of local stresses on the fiber architecture, like Refs. [24] and [25] for the left ventricle, might rather express dependence on the actual mathematical model used. However, this dependence not only affects error estimates for material properties but also highly influences numerical stability as pointed out by Duong [26].

Numerical stability depends on a multitude of factors, starting off from the physics through the actual solver scheme to the the mesh quality. Controlling all these influences, and factoring out under which conditions instabilities are a major concern, is difficult. Instead of controlling the quality of a simulation through mesh size and error tolerance we focus on the influence of the order to which dispersion is captured in a given model. Thus, we focus on a scenario that reveals checkerboard instabilities for a dispersion-free model. Although the scenario, demonstrated below, is rather specific, its key features are applicable to a wide range of problems.

To compare the stability of different models, we match them to the same loading protocol. Next, we identify another loading condition, which displays directional sensitivity. Finally, we construct a simulation that is dominantly governed by the former protocol, yet is superposed with the latter. As shown in Fig. 1(b), both the HO and 0GST model, show strong directional sensitivity with respect to shear load. Thus, we match biaxial load and simulate a monoaxial setup, as depicted in Fig. 6, which exerts increased shear due to its different constituent materials A and B. Material B is governed by an isotropic Neo-Hookean strain energy density

$$\Psi^B_{\text{isovol}} = C_{\text{Hook}}\overline{\mathbf{E}} : \mathbb{I}, \tag{20}$$

with material coefficient C_{Hook} together with the shape of B chosen such that, during tensile loading, torque is exerted. Material A on the other hand is a ground matrix-fiber composite, following the constitutive law

$$\Psi^A_{\text{isovol}} = \frac{a}{2b} e^{4b\overline{\mathbf{E}}:\mathbb{I}} + \Psi^\mu_f(\overline{\mathbf{E}}), \tag{21}$$

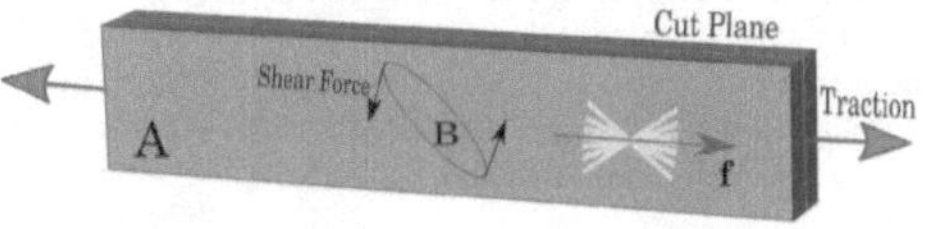

FIG. 6. A beam, composed of two different materials A and B, is subject to monoaxial stretching. Material A consists of fibers with mean direction pointing along **f**, supported by a soft isotropic ground matrix. Material B on the other hand is purely isotropic and chosen to be stiff enough to give rise to strong shear forces (cf. Table II). Lines in magenta show the cut plane used for visualization.

with the different models $\mu \in$ {HO,0GST,2SGST}. In simulation, it is easiest to comply closely with incompressibility by employing a volumetric strain energy $\Psi_{\text{vol}}(J)$ to penalize volume changes. Here we chose [27]

$$\Psi_{\text{vol}} = \Gamma[(J^2-1)/2 - \log J], \tag{22}$$

with bulk modulus $\Gamma = 100$ MPa. The total energy density

$$\Psi^{A/B}_{\text{tot}} = \Psi_{\text{vol}}(J) + \Psi^{A/B}_{\text{isovol}}(\overline{\mathbf{E}}), \tag{23}$$

then, leads to Cauchy stress

$$\boldsymbol{\sigma}^\mu = \mathbf{F}\frac{\partial \Psi^{A/B}_{\text{tot}}}{\partial \mathbf{E}}\mathbf{F}^T \tag{24}$$

and von Mises stress

$$(\sigma^\mu_{\text{Mises}})^2 = \frac{3}{2}\left\{\text{Tr}[(\boldsymbol{\sigma}^\mu)^2] - \text{Tr}^2(\boldsymbol{\sigma}^\mu)\right\}. \tag{25}$$

Parameters for the different isovolumetric energies of material A are listed in Table II and are used together with $C_{\text{Hook}} = 40$ MPa. These parameters are obtained from minimizing the Chi square

$$\chi^2_\mu = \sum_{\tau\in\mathbb{T}_{\text{equi}}}\sum_{i=0}^{N}\left[\sigma^\mu_\tau(1+i\Delta\gamma) - \sigma^{\text{2SGST}}_\tau(1+i\Delta\gamma)\right]^2 \tag{26}$$

for the two equibiaxial stresses $\mathbb{T}_{\text{equi}} = \{(ff, 0^\circ, 1), (n_1n_1, 0^\circ, 1)\}$ with corresponding discretized stretches $\Delta\gamma = 0.22/N$ and $N = 22$. The relative difference

$$\delta^\mu(\gamma) = \left|\frac{\sigma^\mu_\tau - \sigma^{\text{2SGST}}_\tau}{\sigma^{\text{2SGST}}_\tau}\right| \tag{27}$$

for the resulting set of parameters is portrayed in Fig. 7(a). If, in contrast, this change of variables is not performed, and, instead, the same set of parameters is used for all three models, directional sensitivity becomes pronounced even more strongly. However, even if equibiaxial loading is matched to high degree, directional sensitivity analysis shows that sensitivity is lowest for the 2SGST. From

TABLE II. Monoaxial stretch parameters, corresponding to Eq. (21) after models are matched for equibiaxial stretch as shown in Fig. 7(a).

Model	a (kPa)	b	a_f (kPa)	b_f	b_ρ
2SGST	1.5	1	7	40	4.5
HO	0.0363	26.9	4.65	38.1	0
0GST	0.0183	24.6	8.82	48.43	4.5

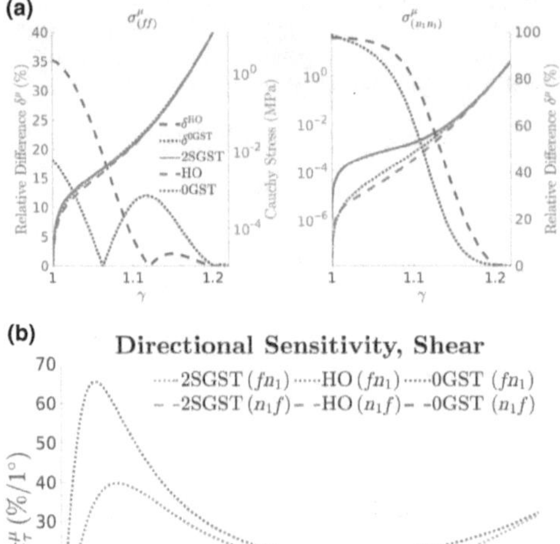

FIG. 7. (a) shows how well the HO and 0GST models match the 2SGST model for equibiaxial stretch after fitting. Corresponding parameters can be found in Table II. True stresses are plotted in blue, whereas relative differences are depicted in purple. (b) Directional sensitivity for the same parameters as in (a) in the case of simple shear.

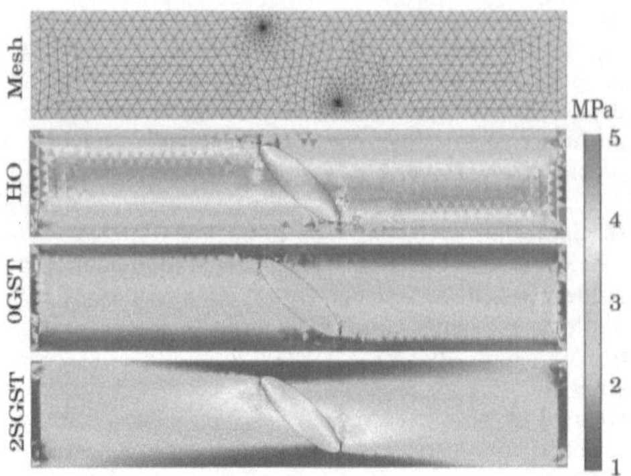

FIG. 8. von Mises stress as defined in Eq. (25) reveals directional instability in monoaxial stretch simulation for the HO, 0GST, and 2SGST models in the cut plane mentioned in Fig. 6. Contrary to the 2SGST model, HO shows a clear checkerboard pattern, which is a namesake for the instability that arises from directional sensitivity. The 0GST model shows intermediate behavior as expected. The result is shown in the reference frame for 18% stretch. The numerical scheme no longer converges for stretches above 19% in the case of HO. In the top subfigure the three-dimensional (3D) mesh projected onto the cut plane is plotted. It should be noted that the checkerboard patterns at the left and right boundaries are due to the numeric scheme. In the case of internal angles below 90° such singularities are a common feature in FEM simulations.

Fig. 7(b) it can be deduced that, for example, at $\gamma = 0.1$ directional sensitivities $\varepsilon^{\mu}_{(fn_1)}$ of the HO and 0GST models are roughly ten times larger than that of the 2SGST model. As shear increases, the relation changes qualitatively and $\varepsilon^{\mathrm{2SGST}}_{(fn_1)} > \varepsilon^{\mathrm{HO}}_{(fn_1)}$, which can be attributed to the strong nonlinearity in isotropic energy ($b = 26.9$). Also the bivariate nature of the 0GST is revealed, approaching $\varepsilon^{\mathrm{2SGST}}_{fn_1}$ on the one hand, and $\varepsilon^{\mathrm{HO}}_{n_1 f}$ on the other hand as γ increases.

Surely this sensitivity alone is not capable of predicting stable or unstable behavior, far and foremost because actual *simple* shear is not present in this simulation. Yet, it nicely motivates the appearance of jigsaw patterns, which can be observed in the von Mises stress defined in Eq. (25) and pictured in Fig. 8. It can be observed that the strength of these patterns decreases from HO, over 0GST to 2SGST. Moreover, the algorithm did not converge for the HO model beyond a stretch of $\gamma - 1 = 19\%$. Also the 0GST model ceased to converge beyond 15% if the ramping is not reduced from 3% to 1% per step. At the same time, the 2SGST showed no irregular behavior for stretches up to 30%. At stretches this large, incompressibility no longer holds with the chosen bulk modulus and the parameters are not fine tuned to match equibiaxial stretch beyond $\gamma - 1 = 22\%$, prohibiting further comparison between the models.

All simulations are performed using COMSOL Multiphysics version 5.4 with FEM solver *PARDISO*, assuring a relative error tolerance of 10^{-3}. Variables to be solved for are fully coupled with an automatic nonlinear Newton method. The mesh contains approximately 20 000 prisms, which, together with cubic serendipidity interpolation functions, amount to a total of approximately 450 000 degrees of freedom. Tensile load is initially ramped by 3% per step, which later gets supplemented by a 1% increase per step as instabilities arise.

VI. DISCUSSION AND CONCLUSIONS

Considering Jensen's inequality sparked the idea to use a squared, instead of linear, GST as an anchor point of the Taylor series of the AI. Convergence analysis, then, shows reduced errors for the SGST models compared to their

GST counterpart of same polynomial order, when considering simple shear and biaxial stretch. As fiber architecture has a strong influence on material mechanics, said analysis contains, both fibers aligned with principle directions of the deformation, as well as fibers rotated by 45° in the respective plane.

Evidently, depending on the extent of deformation, the 2SGST model makes for a reliable substitute of the AI in simulations. Although, in principle, Taylor expansions can be taken to an arbitrary order, since we are dealing with multivariate expressions, they quickly increase in computational costs as demonstrated in Sec. IV. This effect gets weakened by the nSGST models, because the amount of summands does not grow as fast as for the nGST models. Nontheless, if n gets increased, a complementary increase in accuracy is quickly weighed out by computation time. As a result, if better accuracy is needed, the 2SGST, instead, might be used in conjunction with additive decomposition of the fiber density ρ as detailed in Refs. [7] and [28]. Consequently, also nonaffine deformations, crimping and buckling [29,30] or reorientation [31] of fibers, can be included, which is by default not possible for an approach using Taylor series only.

Sensitivity analysis, on the other hand, reveals how dispersion models deviate from unidirectional ones. Although Holzapfel *et al.* [13] showed that the 0GST and AI can be matched equally well to equibiaxial and uniaxial experiments on aortic tissue, it becomes evident that these models no longer show the same behavior once fibers are rotated. Further, said sensitivity can lead to checkerboard instabilities during simulation if multiple loading conditions are superposed. A good recipe for instabilities involves strong directional sensitivity, which might be due to a weak ground matrix, plus material inhomogeneities breaking the symmetry of the loading protocol. These conditions can be found, for example, in cardiac tissue involving irregular, infarcted regions, which get even reinforced by strong stresses during systole. Also materials displaying pronounced gradients in their fiber architecture, such as the ventricular heart wall or arteries, might be vulnerable to directional sensitivity.

The advise to use dispersion in order to overcome instabilities is to be taken with a pinch of salt, though, as numerical stability, in principle, should not decide over what kind of physics to implement. Consequently, instead, experiments have to be consulted to rule out the actual directional sensitivity of a given material. This factors in, especially, when quantitative, patient-specific studies are conducted. Further, we want to highlight that simulations are only a viable tool in predicting material behavior, for as long as the loading protocols encountered in computations are validated in experiments. Admittedly, when choosing our model parameters, we violate this key prerequisite, as we consider only biaxial stretch as a reference for the HO, 0GST, and 2SGST model, although in simulation of monoaxial stretch, a convoluted superposition of shear and stretch can be observed. Consequently, different numerical stability and altered stress fields are observed, indicating that a larger set of reference data is needed to properly inform simulation. It has been noted in Ref. [32] that the amount of independent tests, needed to fully describe a material is at least equal to the amount of invariants associated with the material. Since different orders n are associated with qualitatively different nSGST models, we want to remark that even more independent experiments are needed to make an accurate choice of n. If the required amount of independent experiments is not met, we advice to use the model with lowest sensitivity with respect to possible sources of errors, like for example the mean fiber orientation.

We want to emphasize, that, although a specific fiber density, namely the symmetric von Mises distribution, is employed in this work, the principle idea behind SGST models can be extended to other, e.g., nonsymmetric, distributions analogously [20,29,33]. Also cross terms between different fiber families as detailed by Melnik *et al.* [34] show the potential to benefit from an SGST approach.

Characterizing the architecture and orientation of fibers is crucial to predict the mechanical response of soft materials. As the SGST models can be used for fast and robust simulations, they offer likewise robust and noninvasive numerical tool for clinical treatment. One of their applications is to guide patient care in cardiac ischemia. As demonstrated by Fomovsky *et al.* [35,36], fiber architecture is essential when designing therapeutic implants. Our further work focuses on utilization of the SGST models for *in silico* experiments to optimize engineered tissue scaffolds [37,38] and hence instruct personalized solutions for recovering pump function of the patient's heart. Another potential application for SGST models is the estimation of peak stresses, which goes hand in hand with the directional sensitivity of the model of choice. Consequently, this choice must be made with care, for example, in the analysis of rupture in aortic aneurysm [39], or atherosclerotic plaque [40]. Likewise, the load-bearing capacity of tendons and ligaments can be studied and optimized [30,41] using the proposed models.

ACKNOWLEDGMENTS

The authors thank Alain Pumir, Wolfram-Hubertus Zimmermann and Gerhard Holzapfel for their advice and fruitful discussions. This work is supported by the Max Planck Society and the German Center for Cardiovascular Research.

APPENDIX: STRUCTURE-TENSOR COMPONENTS

All structure tensors necessary to calculate either nGST to fourth, or the nSGST to second order, are listed below.

Due to the transversely isotropic nature of a rotationally symmetric fiber family, the following notation is used, where f denotes the fiber direction while n_1 and n_2 express two arbitrary normal directions. Due to this symmetry, directions n_1 and n_2 can be used interchangeably. Further, it holds that all tensors listed below exert the highest degree of symmetry, meaning that they remain unchanged under any permutation of indices, wherefore only the amount of occurrences (i, j, k) is accounted for, employing the style (f^i, n_1^j, n_2^k). All components not listed are zero.

To further simplify notation, we define the ith tensorial power of an arbitrary tensor $\mathbf{A}$ as

$$\mathbf{A}^{\textcircled{i}} = \underbrace{\mathbf{A} \otimes \ldots \otimes \mathbf{A}}_{i \text{ times}}. \tag{A1}$$

1. Fourth order

The components have been derived previously by Pandolfi *et al.* [11] and are as follows:

$$\langle \mathbf{M}^{\textcircled{2}} \rangle = \begin{cases} 1 - 4\kappa + \kappa_2 & \hat{=} (f^4) \\ \dfrac{2\kappa - \kappa_2}{2} & \hat{=} (f^2, n_1^2) \\ \dfrac{3\kappa_2}{8} & \hat{=} (n_1^4) \\ \dfrac{\kappa_2}{8} & \hat{=} (n_1^2, n_2^2). \end{cases} \tag{A2}$$

2. Sixth order

$$\langle \mathbf{M}^{\textcircled{3}} \rangle = \begin{cases} 1 - 6\kappa + 3\kappa_2 - \kappa_3 & \hat{=} (f^6) \\ \dfrac{\kappa_3}{2} + \kappa - \kappa_2 & \hat{=} (f^4, n_1^2) \\ 3\dfrac{\kappa_2 - \kappa_3}{8} & \hat{=} (f^2, n_1^4) \\ \dfrac{\kappa_2 - \kappa_3}{8} & \hat{=} (f^2, n_1^2, n_2^2) \\ \dfrac{5\kappa_3}{16} & \hat{=} (n_1^6) \\ \dfrac{\kappa_3}{16} & \hat{=} (n_1^4, n_2^2). \end{cases} \tag{A3}$$

3. Eighth order

$$\langle \mathbf{M}^{\textcircled{4}} \rangle = \begin{cases} 1 - 8\kappa + 6\kappa_2 - 4\kappa_3 + \kappa_4 & \hat{=} (f^8) \\ \dfrac{1}{2}(2\kappa - 3\kappa_2 + 3\kappa_3 - \kappa_4) & \hat{=} (f^6, n_1^2) \\ \dfrac{3}{8}(\kappa_4 - 2\kappa_3 + \kappa_2) & \hat{=} (f^4, n_1^4) \\ \dfrac{1}{8}(\kappa_4 - 2\kappa_3 + \kappa_2) & \hat{=} (f^4, n_1^2, n_2^2) \\ \dfrac{5}{16}(\kappa_3 - \kappa_4) & \hat{=} (f^2, n_1^6) \\ \dfrac{1}{16}(\kappa_3 - \kappa_4) & \hat{=} (f^2, n_1^4, n_2^2) \\ \dfrac{35}{128}\kappa_4 & \hat{=} (n_1^8) \\ \dfrac{5}{128}\kappa_4 & \hat{=} (n_1^6, n_2^2) \\ \dfrac{3}{128}\kappa_4 & \hat{=} (n_1^4, n_2^4). \end{cases} \tag{A4}$$

4. Different coefficients κ_i

Generally, we define

$$\kappa = \frac{1}{2}\langle \sin^2 \Theta \rangle \quad \text{and} \quad \kappa_i = \langle \sin^{2i} \Theta \rangle.$$

It follows straight forward that

$$\begin{aligned} \kappa &= \frac{1}{2} + \frac{1}{8b_\rho} - \frac{1}{\sqrt{8\pi b_\rho}} \frac{e^{2b_\rho}}{\operatorname{erfi}(\sqrt{2b_\rho})} && \xrightarrow{b_\rho \to 0} \frac{1}{3} \\ \kappa_2 &= \frac{3\kappa - 1}{2b_\rho} + 2\kappa && \xrightarrow{b_\rho \to 0} \frac{8}{15} \\ \kappa_3 &= \frac{5\kappa_2 - 14\kappa + 2}{4b_\rho} + 2(\kappa_2 - \kappa) && \xrightarrow{b_\rho \to 0} \frac{16}{35} \\ \kappa_4 &= \frac{7\kappa_3 - 16\kappa_2 + 22\kappa - 2}{4b_\rho} \\ &\quad + 3(\kappa_3 - \kappa_2) + 2\kappa && \xrightarrow{b_\rho \to 0} \frac{128}{315}. \end{aligned} \tag{A5}$$

In the limit $b_\rho \to \infty$ all parameters converge to zero.

[1] P. Savadjiev, G. J. Strijkers, A. J. Bakermans, E. Piuze, S. W. Zucker, and K. Siddiqi, Heart wall myofibers are arranged in minimal surfaces to optimize organ function, Proc. Natl. Acad. Sci. **109**, 9248 (2012).

[2] M. Amabili, P. Balasubramanian, I. Bozzo, I. D. Breslavsky, G. Ferrari, G. Franchini, F. Giovanniello, and C. Pogue, Nonlinear Dynamics of Human Aortas for Material Characterization, Phys. Rev. X **10**, 011015 (2020).

[3] V. Wang, P. Nielsen, and M. Nash, Image-based predictive modeling of heart mechanics, Annu. Rev. Biomed. Eng. **17**, 351 (2015).

[4] P. Lamata, A. Cookson, and N. Smith, Clinical diagnostic biomarkers from the personalization of computational models of cardiac physiology, Ann. Biomed. Eng. **44**, 46 (2016).

[5] M. C. Murphy, D. T. Jones, C. R. Jack, Jr., K. J. Glaser, M. L. Senjem, A. Manduca, J. P. Felmlee, R. E. Carter, R. L. Ehman, and J. Huston III, Regional brain stiffness changes across the Alzheimer's disease spectrum, NeuroImage: Clin. **10**, 283 (2016).

[6] T. C. Gasser, R. W. Ogden, and G. A. Holzapfel, Hyperelastic modelling of arterial layers with distributed collagen fibre orientations, J. R. Soc. Interface **3**, 15 (2006).

[7] K. Volokh, On arterial fiber dispersion and auxetic effect, J. Biomech. **61**, 123 (2017).

[8] Y. Lanir, Constitutive equations for fibrous connective tissues, J. Biomech. **16**, 1 (1983).

[9] G. A. Holzapfel and R. W. Ogden, On fiber dispersion models: Exclusion of compressed fibers and spurious model comparisons, J. Elast. **129**, 49 (2017).

[10] Y. Lanir and R. Namani, Reliability of structure tensors in representing soft tissues structure, J. Mech. Behav. Biomed. Mater. **46**, 222 (2015).

[11] A. Pandolfi and M. Vasta, Fiber distributed hyperelastic modeling of biological tissues, Mech. Mater. **44**, 151 (2012).

[12] D. H. Cortes, S. P. Lake, J. A. Kadlowec, L. J. Soslowsky, and D. M. Elliott, Characterizing the mechanical contribution of fiber angular distribution in connective tissue: Comparison of two modeling approaches, Biomech. Model. Mechanobiol. **9**, 651 (2010).

[13] G. A. Holzapfel, R. W. Ogden, and S. Sherifova, On fibre dispersion modelling of soft biological tissues: A review, Proc. R. Soc. A **475**, 20180736 (2019).

[14] H. Gao, W. G. Li, L. Cai, C. Berry, and X. Y. Luo, Parameter estimation in a Holzapfel–Ogden law for healthy myocardium, J. Eng. Math. **95**, 231 (2015).

[15] O. Gültekin, G. Sommer, and G. A. Holzapfel, An orthotropic viscoelastic model for the passive myocardium: Continuum basis and numerical treatment, Comput. Methods Biomech. Biomed. Eng. **19**, 1647 (2016).

[16] G. A. Holzapfel and R. W. Ogden, Constitutive modelling of passive myocardium: A structurally based framework for material characterization, Philos. Trans. R. Soc. A: Math. Phys. Eng. Sci. **367**, 3445 (2009).

[17] G. A. Holzapfel, T. C. Gasser, and R. W. Ogden, A new constitutive framework for arterial wall mechanics and a comparative study of material models, J. Elast. Phys. Sci. Solids **61**, 1 (2000).

[18] J.-J. Hu, S. Baek, and J. Humphrey, Stress–strain behavior of the passive basilar artery in normotension and hypertension, J. Biomech. **40**, 2559 (2007).

[19] G. Sommer, A. J. Schriefl, M. Andrä, M. Sacherer, C. Viertler, H. Wolinski, and G. A. Holzapfel, Biomechanical properties and microstructure of human ventricular myocardium, Acta Biomater. **24**, 172 (2015).

[20] J. A. Niestrawska, C. Viertler, P. Regitnig, T. U. Cohnert, G. Sommer, and G. A. Holzapfel, Microstructure and mechanics of healthy and aneurysmatic abdominal aortas: Experimental analysis and modelling, J. R. Soc. Interface **13**, 20160620 (2016).

[21] See Supplemental Material at http://link.aps.org/supplemental/10.1103/PhysRevApplied.13.064039 for MATLAB library comprising algorithms to compute stresses for the *n*GST, *n*SGST, and AI model.

[22] M. S. Sacks, Incorporation of experimentally-derived fiber orientation into a structural constitutive model for planar collagenous tissues, J. Biomech. Eng. **125**, 280 (2003).

[23] T. S. Eriksson, A. J. Prassl, G. Plank, and G. A. Holzapfel, Modeling the dispersion in electromechanically coupled myocardium, Int. J. Numer. Methods Biomed. Eng. **29**, 1267 (2013).

[24] A. Nikou, R. C. Gorman, and J. F. Wenk, Sensitivity of left ventricular mechanics to myofiber architecture: A finite ele-ment study, Proc. Inst. Mech. Eng., Part H: J. Eng. Med. **230**, 594 (2016).

[25] H. M. Wang, H. Gao, X. Y. Luo, C. Berry, B. E. Griffith, R. W. Ogden, and T. J. Wang, Structure-based finite strain modelling of the human left ventricle in diastole, Int. J. Numer. Methods Biomed. Eng. **29**, 83 (2013).

[26] M. T. Duong, Ph.D. book Universitätsbibliothek der RWTH Aachen (2015).

[27] B. Baillargeon, N. Rebelo, D. D. Fox, R. L. Taylor, and E. Kuhl, The living heart project: A robust and integrative simulator for human heart function, Eur. J. Mech., A/Solids **48**, 38 (2014).

[28] K. Li, R. W. Ogden, and G. A. Holzapfel, A discrete fibre dispersion method for excluding fibres under compression in the modelling of fibrous tissues, J. R. Soc. Interface **15**, 20170766 (2018).

[29] H. Weisbecker, M. J. Unterberger, and G. A. Holzapfel, Constitutive modelling of arteries considering fibre recruitment and three-dimensional fibre distribution, J. R. Soc. Interface **12**, 20150111 (2015).

[30] K. M. Hamdia, M. Marino, X. Zhuang, P. Wriggers, and T. Rabczuk, Sensitivity analysis for the mechanics of tendons and ligaments: Investigation on the effects of collagen structural properties via a multiscale modeling approach, Int. J. Numer. Methods Biomed. Eng. **35**, e3209 (2019).

[31] S. P. Lake, D. H. Cortes, J. A. Kadlowec, L. J. Soslowsky, and D. M. Elliott, Evaluation of affine fiber kinematics in human supraspinatus tendon using quantitative projec-tion plot analysis, Biomech. Model. Mechanobiol. **11**, 197 (2012).

[32] G. A. Holzapfel and R. W. Ogden, On planar biaxial tests for anisotropic nonlinearly elastic solids. A continuum mechanical framework, Math. Mech. Solids **14**, 474 (2009).

[33] A. J. Schriefl, G. Zeindlinger, D. M. Pierce, P. Regitnig, and G. A. Holzapfel, Determination of the layer-specific distributed collagen fibre orientations in human thoracic and abdominal aortas and common iliac arteries, J. R. Soc. Interface **9**, 1275 (2011).

[34] A. V. Melnik, X. Luo, and R. W. Ogden, A generalised structure tensor model for the mixed invariant i8, Int. J. Non Linear Mech. **107**, 137 (2018).

[35] G. M. Fomovsky, J. R. Macadangdang, G. Ailawadi, and J. W. Holmes, Model-based design of mechanical therapies

for myocardial infarction, J. Cardiovasc. Transl. Res. **4**, 82 (2011).

[36] G. M. Fomovsky, S. A. Clark, K. M. Parker, G. Ailawadi, and J. W. Holmes, Anisotropic reinforcement of acute anteroapical infarcts improves pump function, Circulation: Heart Failure **5**, 515 (2012).

[37] W.-H. Zimmermann, I. Melnychenko, G. Wasmeier, M. Didié, H. Naito, U. Nixdorff, A. Hess, L. Budinsky, K. Brune, B. Michaelis, S. Dhein, A. Schwoerer, H. Ehmke, and T. Eschenhagen, Engineered heart tissue grafts improve systolic and diastolic function in infarcted rat hearts, Nat. Med. **12**, 452 (2006).

[38] L. Ye, W.-H. Zimmermann, D. J. Garry, and J. Zhang, Patching the heart: Cardiac repair from within and outside, Circ. Res. **113**, 922 (2013).

[39] P. Erhart, J. Roy, J.-P. P. de Vries, M. L. Liljeqvist, C. Grond-Ginsbach, A. Hyhlik-Dürr, and D. Böckler, Prediction of rupture sites in abdominal aortic aneurysms after finite element analysis, J. Endovasc. Ther. **23**, 115 (2016).

[40] N. Maldonado, A. Kelly-Arnold, Y. Vengrenyuk, D. Laudier, J. T. Fallon, R. Virmani, L. Cardoso, and S. Weinbaum, A mechanistic analysis of the role of microcalcifications in atherosclerotic plaque stability: Potential implications for plaque rupture, Am. J. Physiol.: Heart Circ. Physiol. **303**, H619 (2012).

[41] C. K. Kuo, J. E. Marturano, and R. S. Tuan, Novel strategies in tendon and ligament tissue engineering: Advanced biomaterials and regeneration motifs, BMC Sports Sci. Med. Rehabil. **2**, 20 (2010).

3.3 Further Investigations

Although the squared generalized structure tensor (SGST) is discussed to great detail in the paper, a few points remained untouched so far, which are covered in the following section. First, I discuss shortly the plausibility of the results of some calculations directly linked to the SGST. Second, possible advances of the SGST, which did not have room in the paper, are examined. The notation in the following section is adopted from the paper.

3.3.1 Checks and Balances

Given the case that we worked faultlessly, surely, all calculations leading to the SGST model together with the corresponding numerical evaluations are correct. But as experience teaches us the naivety of this assumption, in the following I present some tests used to validate the calculations.

Before diving into the calculations, let me introduce the notation used for the contraction of two tensors **A** and **B** with respective ranks $m > n$, given by

$$(\mathbf{A} \odot \mathbf{B})_{i_1 \dots i_{m-n-1}} = \mathbf{A}_{i_1 \dots i_{m-n} j_1 \dots j_n} \mathbf{B}_{j_1 \dots j_n}, \tag{3.1}$$

where the *Einstein notation* is employed. Regardless whether $m > n$ or *vice versa*, contraction implicitly is always performed for the inner indices and in the case of $m = n$ the result is a scalar.

The full Taylor series expansion was performed using the technical computing software *Mathematica* [127], which offers a large range of tools to perform analytical calculations. Further investigations involving *Matlab* and *COMSOL* are based on these results, thus mandating the disclosure of any flaws in the process. A thorough description of the *Mathematica* codes related to the computation of these Taylor series components can be found in Appendix C.

In order to check whether the analytics or implementation might be wrong, the results from *Mathematica* can be compared to handmade calculations. This is feasible at least for the lower rank tensors appearing in the expansion, that can be found in the appendix of the paper and are supplemented with the corresponding derivations in Appendix B. Since these results are defined with respect to the structure coefficients κ and κ_i, they can be written down in a much more concise manner than the direct representation formulated by *Mathematica* which is demonstrated exemplary by the first component of the SGST

$$\begin{aligned}(\mathbf{H_2})_{f^4} &= \frac{1}{16\sqrt{2\pi}} \frac{4\sqrt{b_\rho}(4b_\rho - 3)\exp(2b_\rho) + 3\sqrt{2\pi}\mathrm{erfi}(\sqrt{2b_\rho}}{\mathrm{erfi}(\sqrt{2b_\rho})} \\ &= 1 - 4\kappa + \kappa_2. \end{aligned} \tag{3.2}$$

Using the structure coefficients defined in an iterative fashion also unveils directly their limit value. Since the coefficients have to stay finite, it can be concluded from Eqs. B.3, B.4a, and B.4b that for $b_\rho \to 0$

$$3\kappa - 1 = 5\kappa_2 - 14\kappa + 2 = 7\kappa_3 - 16\kappa_2 + 22\kappa - 2 = 0$$

holds. Expectedly, these results overlap with those computed by *Mathematica*. Using Eq. B.8, the general rule, which holds $\forall n \in \mathbb{N}\backslash\{1\}$, can be derived, reading

$$\sum_{i=0}^{n-1}(-1)^i\kappa_i\left[(2n-3)\binom{n-2}{i}-(2n-1)\binom{n-1}{i}\right]=0, \tag{3.3}$$

where $\kappa_0 = 1$ and $\kappa_1 = \kappa$. For this equation to make sense, the definition

$$\binom{k}{l}=0, \tag{3.4}$$

given that $l > k$, is employed.

The test given by Eq. 3.3 only checks for correct implementation in *Mathematica*, but plausibility of the analytics themselves also needs clarification. It can be tested against a simple deformation for which the result is known even without any advanced calculation. Because residual stresses are not considered, it is evident that for the choice $\mathbf{C} = \mathbb{I}$ the internal energy vanishes, leaving us with

$$\mathbb{I}^{\textcircled{j}} \odot \left\langle(\mathbf{M}-\langle\mathbf{M}\rangle)^{\textcircled{j}}\right\rangle = \left\langle(\underbrace{\mathbb{I}:\mathbf{M}}_{=1}-\underbrace{\mathbb{I}:\langle\mathbf{M}\rangle}_{=1})^j\right\rangle = 0, \tag{3.5}$$

where the equality $\mathbf{C}^{\textcircled{j}} \odot \mathbf{M}^{\textcircled{j}} = (\mathbf{C}:\mathbf{M})^j$ is used, which holds for all second-rank tensors $\mathbf{C}$ and $\mathbf{M}$. The relationship given by Eq. 3.5 hands us another check for the implementation individual powers, reading

$$\mathbb{I}^{\textcircled{2}} \odot \langle\mathbf{M}^{\textcircled{2}}\rangle = M_{f^4} + 4M_{f^2n_1^2} + 2M_{n_1^2n_2^2} + 2M_{n_1^4} = 1 \tag{3.6a}$$

$$\mathbb{I}^{\textcircled{3}} \odot \langle\mathbf{M}^{\textcircled{3}}\rangle = M_{f^6} + 6(M_{f^4n_1^2} + M_{f^2n_1^4} + M_{f^2n_1^2n_2^2} + M_{n_1^4n_2^2}) = 1 \tag{3.6b}$$

$$\begin{aligned}\mathbb{I}^{\textcircled{4}} \odot \langle\mathbf{M}^{\textcircled{4}}\rangle = {} & M_{f^8} + 8M_{f^6n_1^2} + 12(M_{f^4n_1^4} + M_{f^4n_1^2n_2^2}) \\ & +8M_{f^2n_1^6} + 24M_{f^2n_1^4n_2^2} + 2M_{n_1^8} + 8M_{n_1^6n_2^2} + 6M_{n_1^4n_2^4} = 1.\end{aligned} \tag{3.6c}$$

Inserting the different tensor components given in Eq. A1, A2, and A3 of Ref. [49] yields the correct results.

3.3.2 Advances

In our publication [49], we introduce a very specific structure tensor, namely the SGST $\mathbf{H_2}$, which is used as an anchor point for the Taylor series approximating the AI model, and yields faster convergence than the generalized structure tensor (GST) models previously used. Yet, we did not show that this is the *best* possible anchor point, showing closest proximity to the target function. On the contrary, it is very unlikely that such an anchor point even exists for the different basic loading protocols introduced in Sec. 2.2.2, let alone any superposition. Hence, I want to stretch that, in principle, any symmetric fourth-rank tensor[3] $\mathbf{D} \in \mathbb{R}^{3\times3\times3\times3}$ is a possible option as an anchor point for the Taylor series. Finding such a polynomial yielding better convergence to the AI, however, is all but trivial. One reason is the large dimensionality of the tensors to be dealt with.

[3] With symmetric, here, it is meant that under any permutation of indices, the corresponding entry of $\mathbf{D}$ stays untouched. This leads to a positive definite tensor, meaning that $\mathbf{A}:\mathbf{D}:\mathbf{A} \geq 0\ \forall$ real-valued second-rank tensors $\mathbf{A}$

This, among other things, can lead to observations that might appear counter-intuitive at first glance. Considering the demonstration function $f = e^{x^2}$ pictured in Fig. 2 of Ref. [49], for example, it appears rather comforting to observe that both, $\langle x \rangle$ and $\langle x^2 \rangle$, lie within the integration bounds [-2,2]. With the tensors $\mathbf{H}$ and $\mathbf{H_2}$, though, such a quality no longer holds. This becomes clear when examining their Euclidean norm[4]

$$||\mathbf{H}||_2^2 = \sum_{i,j} H_{i,j}^2 = 6\kappa^2 - 4\kappa + 1, \tag{3.7a}$$

$$||\mathbf{H_2}||_2^2 = \frac{35}{4}(\kappa_3 - \kappa_4)^2 + 14(2\kappa - 3\kappa_2 + 3\kappa_3 - \kappa_4)^2 + \frac{35\kappa_4^2}{128} + (1 - 8\kappa + 6\kappa_2 - 4\kappa_3 + \kappa_4)^2 + \frac{105}{4}(\kappa_2 - 2\kappa_3 + \kappa_4)^2, \tag{3.7b}$$

$$||\mathbf{M}||_2 = 1. \tag{3.7c}$$

The norm of $\mathbf{M}$, by design, is constant no matter what angle the corresponding fiber has. The other two tensors, in contrast, only meet this value for $b_\rho \to \infty$ which is demonstrated in Fig. 3.3. This can be interpreted as such that $\mathbf{M}$ lies on the surface of a high dimensional sphere whereas $||\mathbf{H}||_2$ and $||\mathbf{H_2}||_2$ are confined to the interior with the SGST being closer to the origin.

For different loading protocols, some areas of this high dimensional sphere are affected more strongly than others, hence promoting that tensors closer to such surface areas will show better proximity to the AI. This approach might be of particular interest when including the decomposition of the fiber density into a linear superposition of basis functions as discussed in the paper and used in Ref. [83]. For the individual basis functions, the importance of particular deformations may vary, thus bolstering the use of different structure tensors.

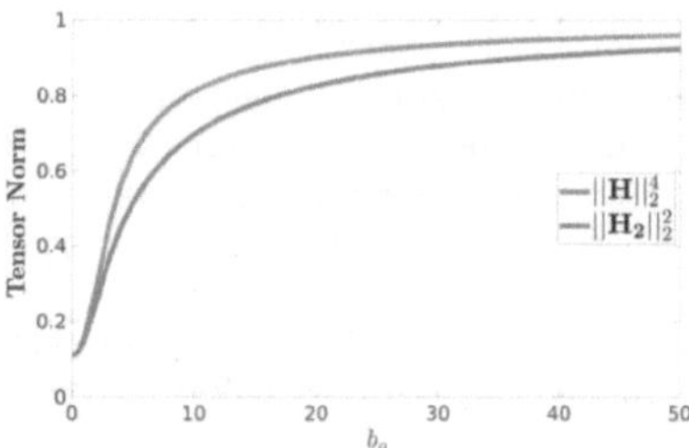

FIGURE 3.3: Euclidian norms of the GST (Eq. 8 Ref. [49]) and SGST (Eq. 13 Ref. [49]). As a means to keep the two norms related to the same vector space it is necessary to square the value for the GST.

In addition to various anchor points that could be used, also various fiber energy densities $\Psi(p(\epsilon))$ are potential candidates for the Taylor series expansion. As long as $p(x)$ is a convex polynomial, Jensen's inequality promises that

$$\langle \Psi(p(\epsilon)) \rangle \geq \Psi(\langle p(\epsilon) \rangle) \geq \Psi(p(\langle \epsilon \rangle)), \tag{3.8}$$

thus advocating to use $\langle p(\epsilon) \rangle$ rather than $\langle \epsilon \rangle$ as an anchor point. This signifies a new paradigm for the approximation of the AI.

[4]There is no particular reason behind this choice. Other norms can do the same trick.

Chapter 4

Successive Ventricular Modeling

As discussed in Sec. 1.2, heart disease is a dominant cause of death especially in the western world. It, thus, comes to no surprise that plenty of medical studies have been performed so as to unravel the cause, nature, and possible treatments of myocardial infarction. With an increased computational power, conjoined with advanced measurement techniques, like MRI simulation-aided studies are also performed. The first model describes the left ventricle as spherical pressure vessels [133], which I used as an inspiration to derive a structure-based model describing the Klotz curve in Sec. 2.4. Some authors go even as far as to reduce the heart to a thin membrane [14], but it has been found that for heterogeneous materials, such as an infarcted heart, stresses in the border zone between the different constituents cannot be captured adequately this way. Other authors, in contrast, depict the left ventricle as an infinitely long cylinder in an effort to analyze transmural stress profiles [84]. Idealized ellipsoidal models quickly took over as they resemble the left ventricular geometry more closely [67, 85–88]. With the increasing capacity of MRI also patient-specific reconstructions of the ventricle became more popular [48, 68, 73, 89, 90]. Usually, a snapshot of the heart at early diastole, where total stresses are the lowest, is used for segmentation which helps with the three-dimensional (3D) reconstruction of the geometry. This approach, in turn, gets augmented, nowadays, by algorithms seeking to find the truly unloaded state of the heart/ventricle [47, 91].

Standing on the shoulders of giants, of course, it is tempting to simply adopt the most recent models in cardiovascular mechanics research and make new findings from there on. However, these models encompass a plethora of different variables, manifest in the geometry, heart architecture, constitutive model, and external loadings, like e.g. the ESV. Hence, when studying the design of a new EHM graft, it can be expedient to repeat some of the steps above, therefore reducing the complexity and amount of variables that allows for a better understanding of the influence of those variables kept. In this chapter, I seek to elucidate the mechanical benefits of an EHM patch that supports an infarcted region in the left ventricle. For that purpose, I first introduce the constitutive laws governing active contraction in Sec. 4.1. In the next step, the EHM is investigated just by itself in Sec. 4.2.1, which is used to learn how shape and size influence the capacity to exert pressure on the underlying tissue. In Sec. 4.2.2, a transversely isotropic spherical model of the left ventricle supplements the interaction between infarct and EHM. Finally, the previous results are used in Sec. 4.3.1 to guide the modeling of an elliptical ventricle which displays a realistic fiber architecture incorporating also fiber dispersion. This step is aimed at validating the results of the spherical model, plus furthering our understanding of how the fiber architecture influences EHM capacity.

4.1 Active Myocardium

Undoubtedly, a key feature of muscularized tissue is its ability to actively contract after receiving a corresponding stimulus. The transmission of said stimulus gives rise to complex and somewhat mesmerizing electro-chemical dynamics which, upon malfunction, can trigger a cascade of events, causing atrial fibrillation which is associated with an increased risk for the very MI we seek to heal [92]. However, in this work, signal propagation is completely omitted for the benefit of mechanical tissue response. In essence, this means that the electrical stimulus acts simultaneously in the entire tissue without any delays, which is justified by its rapid propagation.

In Sec. 1.1.2 the Frank-Starling mechanism, often paraphrased as "the heart pumps what it gets", was introduced. This increased ejection volume is only possible through an raise in contractile performance of the cardiomyocytes. It was found in experiments on cardiomyocytes of cats [93] and rats [129, 94] that the relation between extension and tension is linear. Based on these findings, *Tözeren* formulated a linear stress-strain relation, where the stress is expressed in terms of the Cauchy stress [95]. It is important to note here that the aforementioned experiments show a linear force-length relationship which results in a linear first Piola-Kirchoff stress tensor as defined in Eq. 2.18 as opposed to a linear Cauchy stress. Nonetheless, the linear active Cauchy stress model

$$T_0 = T_a(1 + \beta_0(\lambda - 1)) \tag{4.1}$$

became popular in simulations involving the entire beating cycle [17, 48, 84, 96, 97] as, in addition to the stress-strain relation, the author also provides a calcium-based bridge to electrophysiology. A cross-species study found a set of optimal model parameters for Eq. 4.1 which take the values $T_a = 125\,\text{kPa}$ and $\beta_0 = 1.45$ [96]. Additionally, it was also clarified that the linear law is only well suited for less than fully activated sarcomeres. This finding gets supplemented by another publication [16] suggesting that the length-tension relationship is nonlinear of the form

$$F_{\text{fiber}} = a(\lambda - \lambda_0)^c, \tag{4.2}$$

where F_{fiber} is the tensile force, λ is the sarcomere length and a, c, and λ_0 are fit parameters of which the latter represents the minimal sarcomere length under contraction, as depicted in Fig. 1.4. The authors found exponents c between 0.52 and 2.37, thus clearly advocating the use of a nonlinear model (as e.g. in [98]).

A simple way to incorporate active stresses into a constitutive equation is by simply adding them to the passive stresses

$$\boldsymbol{\sigma}_{\text{tot}} = \boldsymbol{\sigma}_{\text{passive}} + \boldsymbol{\sigma}_{\text{act}}, \tag{4.3}$$

where the active stress takes the form

$$\boldsymbol{\sigma}_{\text{act}} = T_0 \mathbf{F} \mathbf{H}_a \mathbf{F}^T \tag{4.4}$$

with a structure tensor $\mathbf{H}_a$ representing the underlying fiber architecture and T_0 given by Eq. 4.1. Different choices for this structure tensor can be found in Tab. 4.1. They can take a simple form as in example (1) with $\nu = 0$ which relates to the fiber structure in the HO model concerned with their passive deformation. However, as shown in Ref. [49] dispersion can significantly alter the mechanics of fibrous tissue. Although not necessarily derived from an AI, dispersion is manifested in a choice $\nu \neq 0$ for any

(1) $\mathbf{H}_a = \mathbf{f}_0 \otimes \mathbf{f}_0 + \nu \mathbf{s}_0 \otimes \mathbf{s}_0$	$\nu = 0$[99], $\nu = 0.4$[68], $\nu = 0.07$ (healthy)/0.14 (MI)[60]
(2) $\mathbf{H}_a = \mathbf{f}_0 \otimes \mathbf{f}_0 + \nu(\mathbb{I} - \mathbf{f}_0 \otimes \mathbf{f}_0)$	$\nu = 0.2$[100]
(3) $\mathbf{H}_a = \frac{1}{I_{4f}^2}[\mathbf{f}_0 \otimes \mathbf{f}_0 + I_{4f}\nu(\frac{1}{I_{4s}}\mathbf{s}_0 \otimes \mathbf{s}_0 + \frac{1}{I_{4n}}\mathbf{n}_0 \otimes \mathbf{n}_0)]$	$\nu = 0.3$[88], $\nu = 0$ [48]

TABLE 4.1: Comparison of different fiber structure tensors used for active contraction. As defined in Sec. 2.1, the orthonormal base system $\mathbf{f}_0, \mathbf{s}_0, \mathbf{n}_0$ represents the fiber, sheet and normal direction in the reference configuration. Choosing values $\nu \gtrsim 0$ pays tribute to the dispersed nature of cardiomyocytes. The length measure I_{4i} with $i \in \{f, s, n\}$ is defined in Eq. 2.5.

example given in Tab. 4.1.

An appropriate choice, both for the active stress T_0 and the structure tensor $\mathbf{H}_a$, has to be made in the context of an application. For the active stress, I choose to invoke a linear force-length relation, that respects the minimal sarcomere length $l_0 = 1.58\mu$m [16], and shows a linear ESPVR at an EF of 66%, which is in accordance with Ref. [10, 12]. This can be accomplished by the energy density

$$\Psi_{\text{act}} = T_a \lambda \left(\frac{\lambda}{2} - \lambda_0 \right), \tag{4.5}$$

where $\lambda_0 = l_0/l_{\text{R}}$ with a sarcomere rest length of $l_{\text{R}} = 1.85\mu$m [99] and

$$\lambda^2 = \mathbf{C} : \mathbf{H}_a. \tag{4.6}$$

This rule can be augmented easily to account for residual stresses by allowing the sarcomere rest length l_{R} to vary regionally. It has been found in rats that the rest length ranges from $l_{\text{R}} = 1.91\,\mu$m at epicardium to $l_{\text{R}} = 1.78\,\mu$m at endocardium [101]. However, since no residual stresses are considered for the passive myocardium in this work, neither is it included in the description of active myocardium. Besides, estimating residual stresses for the EHM would needlessly complicate the modeling procedure.

Following the definition for the first Piola-Kirchoff stress tensor given in Eq. 2.18 we arrive at

$$\mathbf{P}_{\text{act}} = T_a(\lambda - \lambda_0)\frac{\mathbf{F}\mathbf{H}_a}{\lambda}. \tag{4.7}$$

For the unidirectional structure tensor $\mathbf{H}_a = \mathbf{f}_0 \otimes \mathbf{f}_0$ and uniaxial extension

$$\mathbf{F} = \lambda \mathbf{f}_0 \otimes \mathbf{f}_0 + \frac{1}{\sqrt{\lambda}}(\mathbb{I} - \mathbf{f}_0 \otimes \mathbf{f}_0) \tag{4.8}$$

this translates directly to a linear first (as opposed to second) Piola-Kirchoff stress

$$(\mathbf{P}_{\text{act}})_{ff} = T_a(\lambda - \lambda_0), \tag{4.9}$$

where $\lambda = \sqrt{I_{4f}}$ as defined in Eq. 2.5 holds. From here, a Taylor-Series expansion of the AI of Eq. 4.5 about the GST

$$\mathbf{H} = \kappa \mathbb{I} + (1 - 3\kappa)\mathbf{f}_0 \otimes \mathbf{f}_0 \tag{4.10}$$

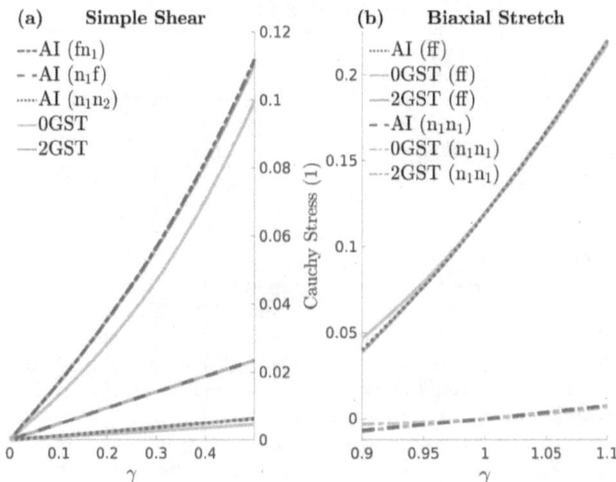

FIGURE 4.1: Showcases for the accuracy with which the 0GST and 2GST model approximate the AI of $\Psi_{\mathbf{act}}$ (see Eq. 4.5). Since it is just a linear pre-factor w.l.o.g. $T_a = 1$ can be chosen. (a) Cauchy stress under simple shear. (b) Cauchy stress under biaxial tensile load. Respective deformation protocols can be found in Sec. 2.2.2. In both cases, the 2GST model shows strong accordance with the AI model.

as introduced in Ref. [49] can be performed, which yields (for a detailed calculation please see Appendix D)

$$\Psi_{\text{act}}^{\text{0GST}} = T_a \left(\frac{1}{2}\lambda^2 - \lambda_0 \lambda \right) \tag{4.11a}$$

$$\Psi_{\text{act}}^{\text{2GST}} = T_a \left(\frac{1}{2}\lambda^2 - \lambda_0 \left[\lambda - \frac{1}{8\lambda^3} \mathbf{C}^{②} \odot \left\{ \langle \mathbf{M}^{②} \rangle - \mathbf{H}_a^{②} \right\} \right] \right). \tag{4.11b}$$

Please note that, although equations 4.11a and 4.5 look identical, they are different as the stretch measure λ is defined using different structure tensors. The accuracy to which the two different GST models approximate the AI model is demonstrated in Fig. 4.1. These results justify the use of Eq. 4.11b for the simulation of an idealized, elliptical left ventricle as later described in Sec. 4.3.1.

In the simpler case of a transmurally isotropic sphere, analyzed in Sec. 4.2, the energy density given in Eq. 4.5 is calculated with the structure tensor

$$\mathbf{H}_a = \mathbb{I} - \mathbf{e}_r \otimes \mathbf{e}_r. \tag{4.12}$$

The normalized base vector $\mathbf{e}_r$ points in transmural (radial) direction.

4.2 Geometrical Aspects of EHM patches

4.2.1 Disk Shaped EHM

The question sought to be answered in this section is to find out which geometric arrangement of the EHM promotes pressure generation most efficiently. For that purpose, I consider solely a single slab of artificial tissue undergoing "typical systolic deformations" and compute the resulting stresses exerted on an imaginary heart lying underneath. When taking a look at Fig. 4.2 the phrase "typical systolic deformation" can be understood as a contraction yielding physiological EF, which I mimic by a radial shrinkage $R \to 0.854R$.

A problem that emerges when suturing additional tissue on top of the heart is that, functionally, it can not be integrated completely. This effect is brought to an extreme when the artificial tissue takes the shape of a curved disk as pictured in Fig. 4.2. If it would be possible to cut out any infarcted tissue and directly replace it with EHM (blue), the tissue would be perfectly integrated into the heart and thus could exert contractile forces to their full extend. Contrary, in the case of a tissue disk "glued" to the surface of the heart (red), connectivity is lowered due to an additional degree of freedom. In the operating room, surely, neither of the extremes occurs, yet I investigate the significance of the effect of a free wall on the resulting traction. With the given setup I measure the strength of the EHM by averaging the absolute value of the surface stresses over a small area $\mathcal{A}$ at the center of the disk, yielding

$$t_{\text{avg}} = \frac{1}{A}\int_{\mathcal{A}} ||\boldsymbol{\sigma}\mathbf{n}||\mathrm{d}a \qquad \text{with} \qquad A = \int_{\mathcal{A}} \mathrm{d}a. \tag{4.13}$$

The surface area $\mathcal{A}$ is defined via an intersection between the EHM disk in the reference configuration and a cone pointing from the origin to the center of the disk. The cone exhibits an opening angle of $\Theta_{\text{cone}} = 16°$ with the EHM surface in the reference configuration.

In the analysis, two different modifications of the geometry are distinguished. In case (I), the opening angle Θ is changed while keeping the thickness Δ constant, whereas in case (II), the opening angle is changed while keeping the tissue volume V_{EHM} constant. This average is chosen as it, both, reduces unphysiological effects of the border zone of the EHM and assures accuracy of a discretized FEM solution, which potentially could feature discontinuities, as discussed in Sec. 2.3.

For the passive tissue behavior, I adopt the constitutive law as described in Sec. 2.4

$$\Psi_{\text{passive}} = \frac{a}{2b}[e^{b(I_1-3)} - 1]. \tag{4.14}$$

For convenience, I assume that the mechanical properties of the EHM are identical to that of healthy myocardium, which, in principle, I mimic by setting the parameters to those of the best fit to the Klotz curve, as presented in Tab. 2.2. When only considering the efficacy of EHM, though, absolute values are of no interest and therefore all stresses and corresponding factors can be normalized such that $a = 1$. Additionally, also spatial dimensions are normalized to account for a hypothetical left ventricle being encapsulated by the EHM which results in an internal radius $R = 1 + \Delta$ with $\Delta = 0.27$ as derived in Sec. 2.4. Geared toward the estimation of uncertainties of the stiffening factor b, two different such values are considered.

The constitutive law governing active contraction is given by combining Eqs. 4.5, 4.6, and 4.12. For a spherical arrangement and together with Eq. 2.40a this amounts

a	case	b	T_a
1	(i)	3.83	76.9
	(ii)	7.66	95.2

TABLE 4.2: Constitutive parameters only considering the disk shaped EHM. Active contractile parameter T_a is chosen such that a full ventricle composed of a tissue with stiffening factor b would yield a 66% ejection fraction.

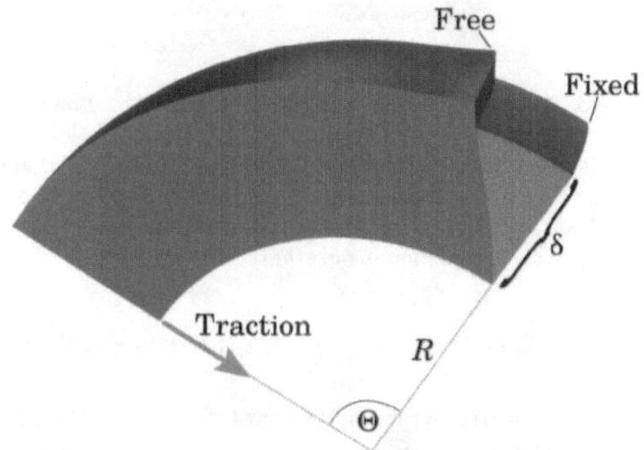

FIGURE 4.2: Slice of the curved EHM disk. Due to rotational symmetry, only a small wedge of the tissue needs to be simulated. In case of a free boundary (red) the additional degree of freedom yields a lowered traction compared with the fixed boundary (blue). Thickness δ and opening angle Θ of the disk are altered between simulations to elucidate how much tissue is needed for an optimal traction force.

to a ventricular pressure of

$$p_a = \int_0^{\Delta} T_a \frac{1 - \frac{\lambda_0}{\sqrt{2}}\sqrt{\lambda_\rho}}{\hat{r}} \mathrm{d}\delta. \tag{4.15}$$

As before, the total energy, and correspondingly the pressure, is obtained from the summation of passive and active terms. This allows adjusting the contractile force coefficient T_a such that with an EDP of 10 and an ESP of 100 a hypothetical left ventricle as described in Sec. 2.4 would yield an EF of 66%. All constitutive parameters used in this section are displayed in Tab. 4.2.

Case (I): Constant Thickness

How efficient is a given EHM patch and what can be considered optimal?

To begin with, let me introduce the term "efficacy", which I define here as the ratio between the actual traction t_{avg}, as defined in Eq. 4.13, and the value a sphere of identical thickness would exert. With this declaration, a blunt answer to the question above would be to say that, regardless of the infarct, covering the entire heart always shows maximal effect because it allows for optimal connectivity of the EHM, plus, simply put, more material exerts more force. Given the aforementioned ingredients,

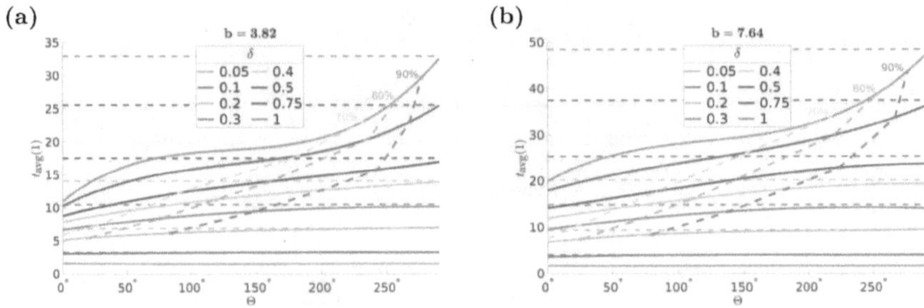

FIGURE 4.3: Average traction as defined in Eq. 4.13 against different opening angles Θ for various thicknesses δ. Dashed, colored lines are corresponding to maximal values a spherical geometry would yield. Gray curves depict for which angle a particular fraction of this value is met (efficiency). (a) and (b) correspond to the two cases (I,*i*) and (I,*ii*) with values presented in Tab. 4.2.

this statement must hold, however, it is worthwhile to examine how precisely additional material influences the effect of the EHM.

In Fig. 4.3 the average traction shows that for small thicknesses $\delta \leq 0.1$ the EHM patch does show maximal efficacy regardless of the opening angle. Implicitly, this means, that adding more material by covering a larger area does not increase the ventricle's capacity to withstand loading pressure. Instead, it is advised to increase the thickness of the patch. This reasoning neglects, of course, that for constant forces, more material sill can deliver more mechanical energy, thus still impacting the pressure-volume relation of the ventricle[1].

Increasing the thickness a bit further reveals that increasing Θ while keeping the efficacy constant necessitates likewise an increase in thickness. This effect is shown separately in Fig. 4.4. Except for the total traction values, the results for the two cases (*i*) and (*ii*) (see Tab. 4.2) do not exhibit any differences noteworthy, thus making the analysis robust against changes in constitutive parameters.

In conclusion, it can be noted that, expectedly, for small thicknesses the effect of a lack of connectivity to the underlying tissue is negligible and other factors should inform how a EHM should be constructed. Starting from a value of roughly $\delta \approx 0.2$, which for $\Delta = 0.2712$ is equivalent to approximately 75% of the myocardial wall thickness, connectivity plays a crucial role in patch design.

Case (II): Constant Volume

Given the total volume of the artificial material, what is the optimal opening angle?

In the case where the total amount of EHM has to be budgeted, maybe due to its costs, it may be of interest to know what the optimal relation between patch thickness and opening angle is. If the volume is kept constant while Θ changes, of course, δ also has to be adjusted as depicted in Fig. 4.5. Among these, the geometry is considered optimal if the average traction given by Eq. 4.13 is at its maximum. The results can be found in Fig. 4.7. Despite $\hat{V}_{\text{EHM}}$ displaying a large range from 5-100% of the interior volume $V_{\text{ref}} = 4\pi R^3/3$ the angles at which the maxima are found are confined

[1] As previously discussed in Sec. 1.1.2, the area encapsulated by the pressure-volume relation equals the total energy consumption per cycle.

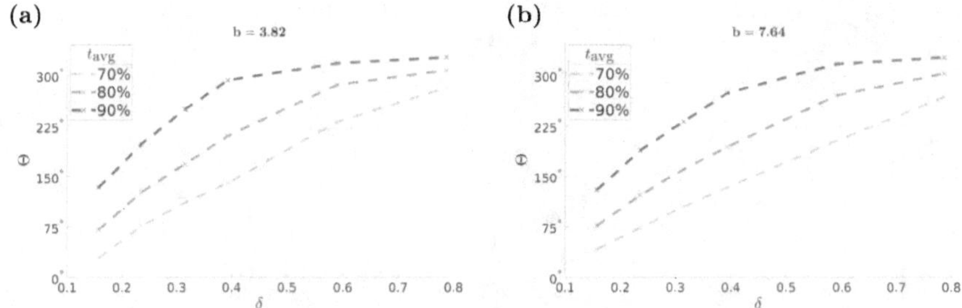

FIGURE 4.4: Curves of constant efficiency for the results presented in Fig. 4.3 with the two different subplots (a) and (b) corresponding to the cases (I,i) and (I,ii) with values presented in Tab. 4.2. The results stay almost untouched by b.

to the interval between $40° - 100°$. This finding is highlighted in Fig. 4.6. It reproduces the previous conclusion that the stiffening parameter b plays only a minor role. Extreme geometries, such as a disk of small volume $\hat{V}_{\mathrm{EHM}} = 0.05$ and large opening angles $\Theta \geq 300°$, amplify numeric inaccuracies which can be observed in Fig. 4.7. However, this is not the reason, all curves in Fig. 4.7 show a little kink for small values of Θ. Instead, this feature arises directly from geometric properties. The same feature can be found when approximating the simulation analytically by roughly guessing the deformation profile. Since using these models to predict the maxima was not crowned with success, they are omitted here.

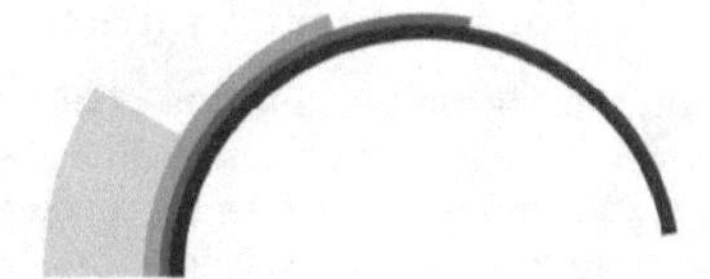

FIGURE 4.5: Profiles of half of the disc with various opening angles while EHM volume is kept constant.

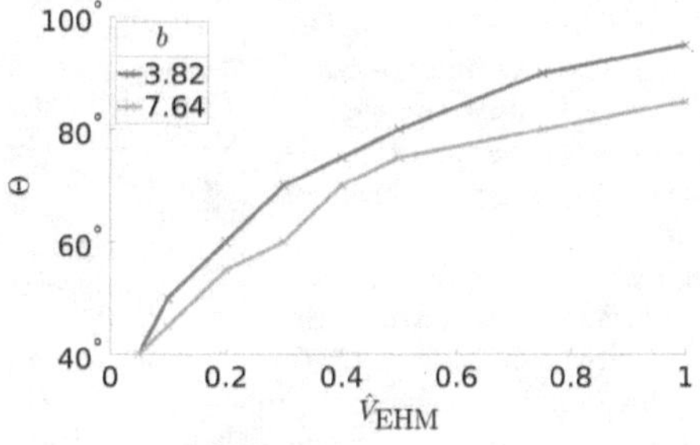

FIGURE 4.6: Parameters for which the average tension t_{avg} from Fig. 4.7 reaches its maximum. The stiffening parameters b expresses only little influence on the slope of the curve.

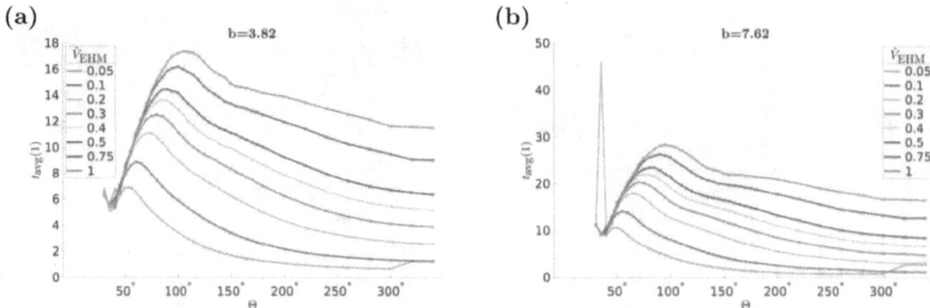

FIGURE 4.7: Average central tensions (E. 4.13) for an EHM of constant normalized volume $\hat{V}_{\text{text}}$ with the two different subplots (a) and (b) corresponding to the cases (II,i) and (II,ii) with values presented in Tab. 4.2. The sharp spike in (b) for $\hat{V}_{\text{EHM}} = 0.2$ and $\Theta \approx 35°$ stems from errors in the simulation. The same holds for the sudden increase beyond $\Theta = 300°$ concerning $\hat{V}_{\text{EHM}} = 0.05$ in both cases, which is due to a poor resolution as the shell becomes extremely thin.

4.2.2 Spherical Left Ventricle

In the previous section, I discussed how the shape of the EHM alone influences its potential to exert force and thus withstand ventricular pressure. In this section, I take the same constitutive laws as in Sec. 4.2.1 and supplement the analysis by a ventricle featuring a scarred domain as depicted in Fig. 4.8. This approach helps to illuminate the interactions between different tissues and further confine previous conclusions.

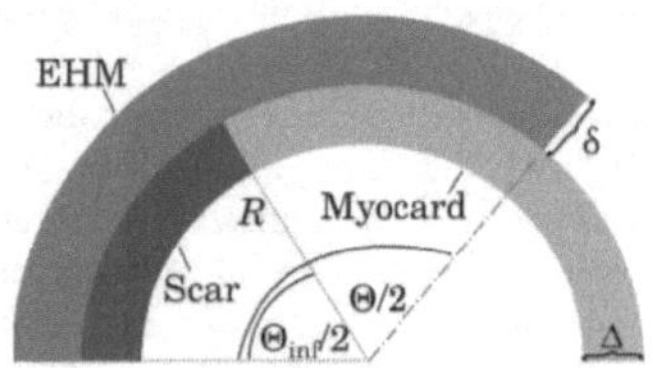

FIGURE 4.8: Halfed cross section of a spherical, infarcted ventricle on which EHM is sutured. Colors represent the three different domains EHM patch, scarred tissue and regular myocardium. The given opening angle of the infarct Θ_{inf} corresponds to an infarction size of 25% with respect to ventricular surface area (induced in Ref. [28]). While Δ is normalized with respect to R, δ is normalized with respect to $R(1 + \Delta)$.

Constitutive model parameters are chosen such that the healthy myocardium, displays the same mechanical properties as the EHM while matching a left ventricle with an EF of 66% in the non-infarcted state. The resultant parameters can be found in Tab. 4.3. Just as before, I analyze the influence of b as well as the EHM size for two different scenarios: (I) constant thickness & (II) constant volume.

Scarred tissue, as described in Sec. 1.2, undergoes several stages of remodeling in which the tissue gets thinned out and structurally strengthened by an increase in collagen content, thus completely changing its mechanical properties. While thinning effectively softens the tissue, the increased collagen content stiffens it. Depending on the age of the infarct, this can lead either to an increased or to decreased left-ventricular EDPVR [24, 26], as previously depicted in Fig. 1.6. To capture this feature I adopt an approach from Ref. [102] where the geometry stays untouched and instead pre-factors in the constitutive law

$$\Psi_{\text{inf}} = \frac{a_{\text{inf}}}{2b}\left[e^{b(I_1-3)} - 1\right] \tag{4.16}$$

are scaled to match with experimental data. Although the authors found an apparent tissue softening factor of roughly 1/2, I want to accommodate the strong variability of scar stiffness, wherefore I include several different constitutive parameters which can be found in Tab. 4.3. Please note that scared tissue does not contain cardiomyocytes, which is why Eq. 4.16 contains only a homogeneous, passive term.

In the Introduction (Sec. 1.2) I discussed the importance of the border zone between scar and healthy myocardium. In simulation contradictory findings were made concerning the importance of explicit modeling of the border zone. In Ref. [99] only a border zone with greatly impaired contractility could reproduce experimentally observed strains while Ref. [103] found the exact opposite, i.e. that making such a functional difference is unnecessary. Because local strains and remodeling are not the focus of this section I decide to use the simple approach of ignoring any functional border zone as reflected by Fig. 4.8.

A critical problem in the simulation of the scarred tissue is that, as it gets compressed by the EHM lying on top, it starts buckling as portrayed in Fig. 4.9. Consequently, incompressibility is violated in the vicinity of the kink and the numerical scheme eventually fails to converge even with the finest mesh resolutions tested. Although buckling amplifies directional sensitivity, switching to a fiber dispersion model does not circumvent poor convergence, wherefore simulations are performed with the simpler model nevertheless. This means, ergo, that not all $\Theta - \delta$ combinations from the previous section are compliant for simulation.

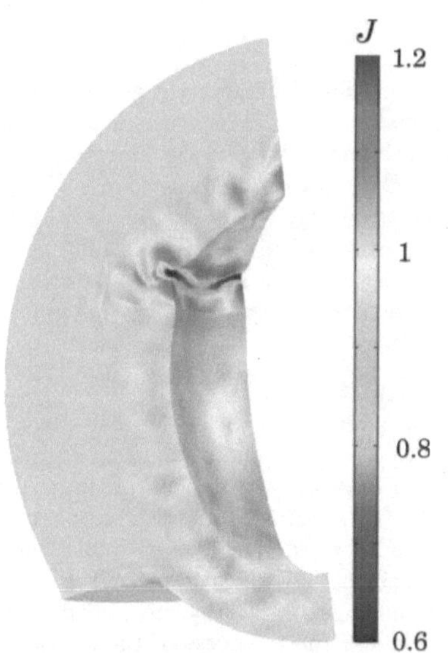

FIGURE 4.9: Slice of the sphere expressing large stresses exerted by a thick EHM causing the non-contractile scar underneath to buckle. This is accompanied by unphysiological volume ratios J (see Eq. 2.10), rendering adequate simulations impossible for large values T_a or δ.

The metrics used to evaluate ventricular performance, derived from pressure-volume relations, typically are Ees, SV, and EF. These I want to complement with a metric combining the SV of the healthy, infarcted and grafted ventricle, hence forming the relative gain in SV (RGSV) which I define as

$$\text{RGSV} = 1 - \frac{\text{SV}_{\text{healthy}} - \text{SV}_{\text{graft}}}{\text{SV}_{\text{healthy}} - \text{SV}_{\text{inf}}}. \tag{4.17}$$

This value is 0 in the infarcted state and increases as EHM is added to the ventricle, eventually exceeding the original SV at values of RGSV>1. The normalized Ees is given by the ratio

$$\nu = \text{Ees}_{\text{graft}}/\text{Ees}_{\text{healthy}} \tag{4.18}$$

of the linear coefficients describing the ESPVR as defined in Eq. 1.2. Loosely speaking, deformations, as portrayed in Fig. 4.9, can be rather irregular wherefore the VV must

a(kPa)	a_{in}	Δ	Θ_{in}	case	b	T_a(kPa)
1.15	$\left(\frac{1}{2}, 1, 3\right) \cdot a$	0.27	120°	(i)	3.82	78.3
				(ii)	7.64	126

TABLE 4.3: Constitutive parameters for a spherical left ventricle that displays an EF of 66% prior to infarction. Passive material properties are related to the findings of Sec. 2.4.

be obtained through integration rather than simple radius identification. Since this volume is not part of the material and thus the simulation domain, instead Gauss law is utilized to transform a volume integral into an integral over the endocardial surface $\partial\mathbb{B}_{\text{endo}}$ yielding

$$\text{VV} = \frac{1}{3}\int_{\partial\mathbb{B}_{\text{endo}}} \mathbf{x}\cdot \mathbf{ds} \tag{4.19}$$

following the same notation as introduced in Sec. 2.1.

In Sec. 1.1.1 it is mentioned that ventricular wall thickening is a key player to achieve large SVs. In the literature, it is claimed that, traditionally, in computer simulation, it can only be accounted for 20% of the 40% wall thickening as fiber sliding is not explicitly targeted [104, 105]. With the simplistic, spherical model described here, a total of 70% wall thickening between diastole and systole can be observed in the healthy state. This follows directly from volume conservation, an EF of 66% and a normalized EDV=2 which stems from the adaption to the Klotz curve.

Case (I): Constant Thickness

Case (I,i): The softer the scar effectively becomes through remodeling, the more severely cardiac pump function is impaired as demonstrated in Fig. 4.10. In fact, during diastole the VV increases due to the infarction but the overall SV, here manifest in the EF, decreases drastically since the ESV increases greatly. As EHM is added to the infarcted ventricle, both EDV and ESV decrease expectedly, thus supporting a regain in SV which eventually exceeds the healthy state. What is alarming at this point is that a thickness coefficient $\delta = 0.05$ is equivalent to an EHM being one fourth the thickness of the myocardium and despite this enormous size it only recovers roughly 40% of the SV at a maximal angle of $\Theta = 360°$. While this clearly is an increase that can decide over life and death it is still telling for how much tissue is actually needed to sustain a healthy cardiac output. How strong incrementing the size of the EHM further impacts cardiac output is estimated using the normalized derivative with respect to volume

$$\Upsilon = \frac{\partial\text{RGSV}}{\partial\hat{V}_{\text{EHM}}} = \frac{\partial\text{RGSV}}{\partial\Theta}\left(\frac{\partial\hat{V}_{\text{EHM}}}{\partial\Theta}\right)^{-1} = \frac{4}{\Delta\hat{V}\sin(\Theta/2)}\frac{\partial\text{RGSV}}{\partial\Theta}, \tag{4.20}$$

where

$$\Delta\hat{V} = (((1+\Delta)\delta + 1 + \Delta)^3 - (1+\Delta)^3) \tag{4.21}$$

is the normalized volume of a full EHM shell. Since an analytic solution to Eq. 4.20 is not available, instead, I use a midpoint finite difference approximation based on the simulation data. The result, displayed in Fig. 4.10e, shows strong similarities to the curves observed for a disk of constant volume (Fig. 4.4). An initial decrease followed by a minimum at 40° leads to a peak at roughly 100° after which EHM impact gradually declines. Both these measures estimate the efficiency of the heart and while Fig. 4.6 displays a small rightward shift in maximal efficiency as EHM thickness increases, the location of the maximum in Fig. 4.10e is virtually independent of δ. A simulation, conducted with a larger scar ($\Theta_{\text{in}} = 144°$ in Fig. 4.11) reveals how the maximal efficiency shifts along with the border zone of the infarct. This advocates an already intuitive assumption that the EHM should cover at least the scarred tissue. Also the inotropy displays only weak responses to an increase in EHM thickness and is mostly dependent on the opening angle.

Varying the scar stiffness alters the absolute values of the individual metrics without qualitatively changing the analysis, as depicted in Fig. E.1 and E.2. Specifically doubling the value of a_{in} from $a/2 \rightarrow a$ shows virtually no changes to the simulation results, whereas a sixfold increase has a small, yet noticeable, impact, thus highlighting the nonlinearity of cardiac mechanics. In effect, scar stiffness plays a minor role in EHM efficiency, wherefore, it appears to be negligible for the design of an optimal EHM patch. Which patient might benefit from an implantation depends on scar stiffness though.

Case (I,*ii*): When increasing the stiffening factor b, the EDV decreases substantially, mandating an increased contractile force in order to keep the same EF. Consequently, buckling, as depicted in Fig. 4.9, is pronounced much more strongly, wherefore the span of thickness parameters for which the simulation shows convergence is reduced. Additionally, the original drop in EF as shown in Fig. 4.12a is not as severe as for the softer tissue, making the ventricle more resilient to infarcts. The combination of a lesser drop in SV and a much stronger contractile force also facilitate the gain in SV shown in Fig. 4.12b. Interestingly, beyond $\Theta = 200°$ additional EHM has nearly no effect in the RGSV at all. The Ees (Fig. 4.12d) on the other hand drops significantly and cannot be recovered with the amount of EHM added here. While for small values Θ the Ees does not show much dependence on the patch thickness, just like in case i, this behavior changes at roughly $\Theta \geq 100°$. Yet, overall changes to the ESPVR stay small.

Case (II): Constant Volume

The analysis of the case where the volume of the EHM patch is kept constant, follows the same lines as done in the previous section. For case (i) the extremal values of the RGSV as shown in Fig. 4.13c, previously observed in the disk model (Fig. 4.6), are extenuated to the point where it is difficult to observe them at all. Instead, the curve quickly plateaus beyond an opening angle of roughly $\Theta \geq 150°$. Only at the largest volumes, the extremal values become significant. This is in great contrast to the findings of case (ii), presented in Fig. 4.14. Here, the extremal values for the RGSV and ESV are clearly visible and while they do not coincide with those shown for the disk (Fig. 4.6) they still show the same trend leading to the conclusion that they form mostly due to the same geometric reasons, i.e. the interplay between connectivity and wall thickness. As with case (I), changing infarct stiffness (see App. E.2) impacts only how efficient the EHM patch is but not what the optimal shape is. With case (ii) EHM buckling plays a crucial role which can be diminished by an increased scar stiffness.

Just like with case (I,i, $a_{\text{inf}} = 0.5a$) the Ees, shown in Fig. 4.13d, is less influenced by the total amount of EHM tissue and instead relies mostly on larger angles Θ. As

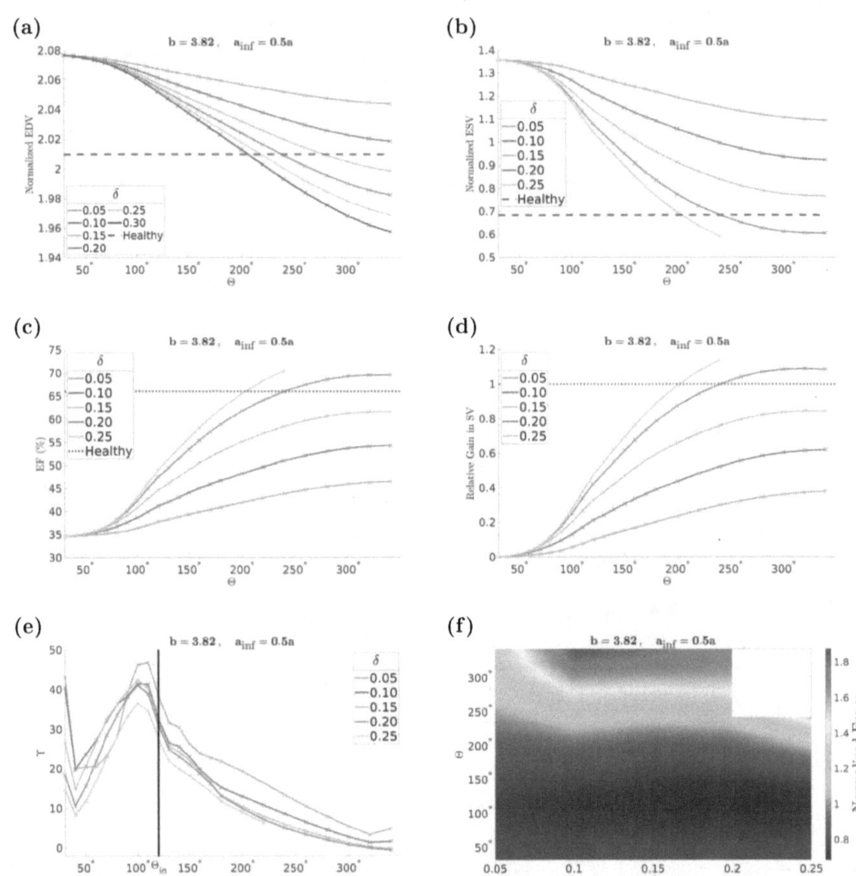

FIGURE 4.10: Case (I,i, $a_{\text{inf}} = 0.5a$) – Changes to the ventricular performance represented by different metrics (a) EDV, (b) ESV, (c) EF, (d) regain in SV (Eq. 4.17), and (f) normalized Ees (Eq. 4.18). While apparent softening of the scarred tissue slightly increases the EDV this effect gets outweighed by the huge increase in ESV thus causing a drop of SV manifesting itself in a lowered EF. Adding EHM increases cardiac output even to a point where it exceeds the SV of a healthy heart. (e) Derivative of RGSV with respect to EHM volume (Eq. 4.20) indicates strong efficacy close to the border zone.

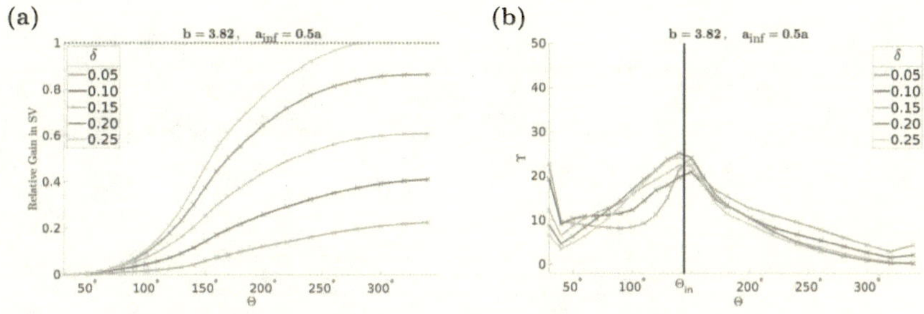

FIGURE 4.11: Case (I,i, $a_{\text{inf}} = 0.5a$) Larger scar $\Theta_{\text{in}} = 144°$ – (a) RGSV (Eq. 4.17) is lowered compared with Fig. 4.10d. (b) Efficiency according to Eq. 4.20 shifts along with the infarct size emphasizing the need to cover the entire infarct.

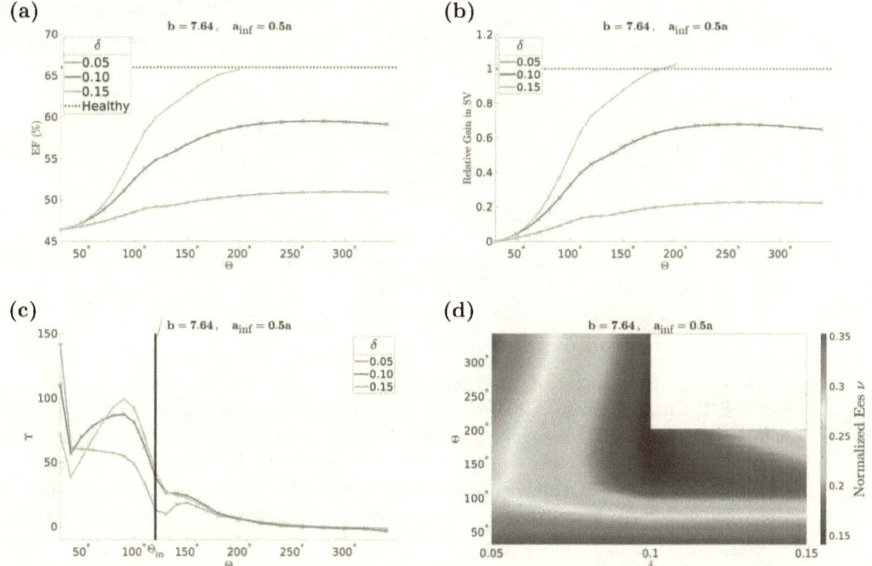

FIGURE 4.12: Case (I,ii, $a_{\text{inf}} = 0.5a$) – Changes to the ventricular performance represented by different metrics (a) regain in SV (Eq. 4.17), (b) EF, and (d) normalized Ees (Eq. 4.18). (c) Derivative of RGSV with respect to EHM volume (Eq. 4.20).The Ees experiences a drastic drop which cannot be recovered by the addition of EHM tissue. Due to the enlarged stiffening coefficient b crimping during systole is amplified wherefore much fewer simulations converge.

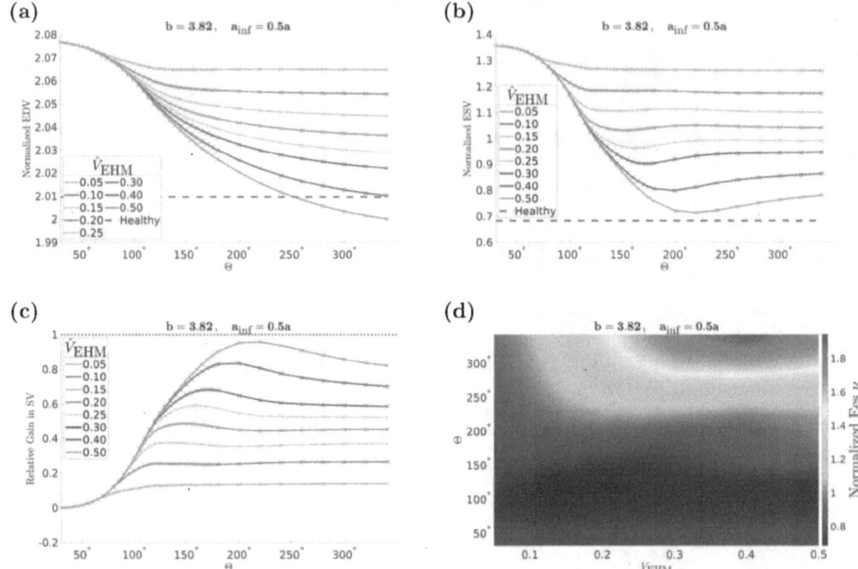

FIGURE 4.13: Case (II,i, $a_{\text{inf}} = 0.5a$) – Changes to the ventricular performance represented by different metrics (a) EDV, (b) ESV, (c) RGSV (Eq. 4.17), and (d) normalized Ees (Eq. 4.18). Extrema, indicating the most efficient EHM distribution, are shallow for small values $\hat{V}_{\text{EHM}}$.

myocardial stiffness is increased, and hence so is the contractile strength of the EHM, inotropy plummets with little to be done for it.

4.2.3 Conclusion & Discussion

In this section, I presented a parameter study highlighting geometric cues for optimal EHM patch design. In the initial Sec. 4.2.1 I focused the attention on how a free boundary and the resulting lack of connectivity impacts the tissues capacity to build up traction forces, which in Sec. 4.2.2 was supplemented with a study on the interaction between myocardium, scar, and patch. The most important conclusions which can be drawn from a comparison of the parameters sets are as follows:

- The intuition that the EHM patch should be larger than the scar is confirmed using the efficiency estimate Υ presented in Figs. 4.10e and 4.11a.
- While traction t_{avg} shows optimal values between $50° \leq \Theta \leq 120°$ for the disk model at constant EHM volume, these values are right shifted for the sphere and depend strongly on the contractile coefficient T_a where smaller such values promote larger opening angles.

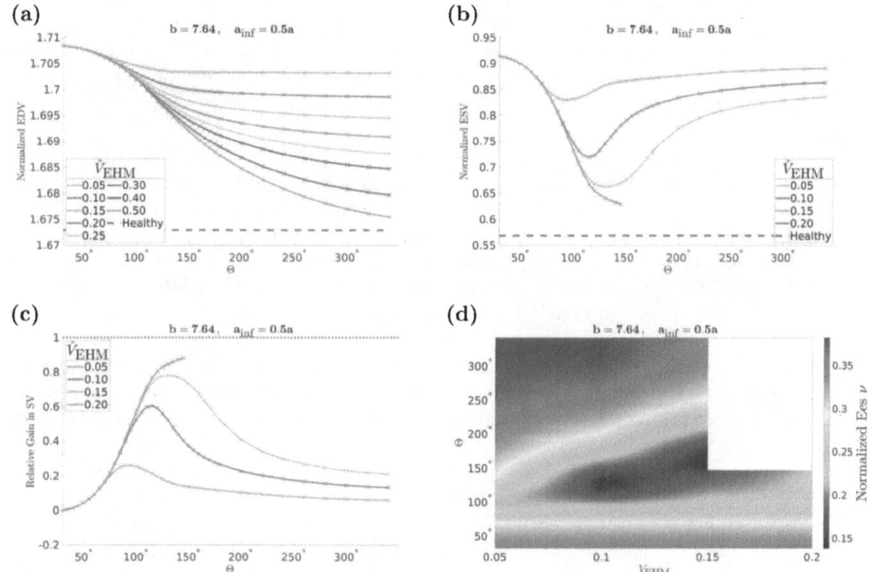

FIGURE 4.14: Case (II,*ii*, $a_{\text{inf}} = 0.5a$) – Changes to the ventricular performance represented by different metrics (a) EDV, (b) ESV, (c) RGSV (Eq. 4.17), and (d) normalized Ees (Eq. 4.18). Extremal values in(b) and (c) are strongly pronounced and right shifted compared with the findings from Fig. 4.6. Just as in Fig. 4.12d the Ees experiences a drastic drop which cannot be recovered by the addition of EHM tissue.

- Also inotropy benefits mostly from larger angles Θ. In case (i) the Ees returns to normal for values roughly $\Theta = 150°$ regardless of scar stiffness.
- For an increased baseline stiffening factor $b = 7.64$ the Ees drops much more drastically and is also much more difficult to recover, indicating the need of patient specific EHM design.
- Scar stiffness a_{inf} does not impact the optimal design of the EHM patch but its total efficiency.
- While doubling the scar stiffness shows barely any impact on the different metrices, increasing it by a sixfold has strong implications. As the myocardium undergoes remodeling over several weeks after the infarct, the exact time point at which EHM tissue is implanted might play a crucial role in its potency as a cure.

This study aimed at obtaining quantitative insights with as little specifications as possible, wherefore normalization is used wherever applicable and also the contractile force is tied to the EF such that is always the same in the respective healthy ventricle. Evidently, such a study is by no means exhaustive and many parameters, like scar size Θ_{inf}, scar stiffening factor b_{inf}, or normalized minimal sarcomere length λ_0, still can be tuned for a better understanding of the models used. Additionally, the parameter space of the patch geometry was probed by just either varying Θ or δ, thus returning two disjoint optimality measures. For a precise and unique solution, an unconstrained variation of the two parameters combined with a cost function for EHM volume could prove to be fruitful. It is discussed in Sec. 1.2 that stresses in the border zone of the scar can cause the infarction to grow. Respecting this effect in the analysis also shows the potential to change some of the results.

Further, future studies must provide evidence, both in simulation and experiment, that the findings made here still hold under more realistic conditions. Especially considering actually thinned scar tissue, or even realistic geometries derived from MRI reconstruction, is of importance to support the claims formulated here.

The following section is dedicated to the understanding of the influence of the fiber architecture in the EHM on its efficiency. For that purpose, the results, presented here, are used to inform what parameters should be used as a base line. A combination of $\Theta = 180°$ and $\delta/\Delta = 0.5$ aims at a reasonable recovery of the SV while keeping the dimensions reasonable with regards to actual implantations. The choice is further supported by the result, that with strong contractile forces also the efficiency measured with Υ (Eq. 4.20) drastically drops above an angle of $\Theta \geq 180°$ rendering additional material ineffective.

In Sec. 4.2.2 it is discussed that buckling of the scarred tissue yields large bulk pressures which are accompanied by increased local strains. These strains spread out, thus leading to a heterogeneous stress distribution at the scar-patch interface bearing the potential of rupture of the already weaker contact. This invokes the question whether, depending on the apparent scar stiffness, there exists a threshold for contractile force which the EHM patch must not cross. If so, it might be beneficial in certain cases to reduce the contractility of the EHM deliberately for the purpose of long-term function preservation.

Paremter	Value	Definition
d	60 mm	Eccentricity
τ	12.5 mm	Basal myocardial wall thickness
$r_{\mathrm{s,endo}}$	23.5 mm	Short inner axis
$r_{\mathrm{l,endo}}$	65 mm	Long inner axis
$r_{\mathrm{s,epi}}$	36 mm	Short outer axis
$r_{\mathrm{l,epi}}$	70 mm	Long outer Axis
λ_{endo}	0.38	First prolate spheroidal coordinate, Endocardium
λ_{epi}	0.57	First prolate spheroidal coordinate, Epicardium

TABLE 4.4: Geometric parameters for prolate-spheroidal left ventricle geometry as proposed by Ref. [67] (and similar to Ref. [86]). Truncation happens at the center along the short axis as depicted in Fig. 4.15 implicating a reference VV $V_0 = 74.5\,\mathrm{mL}$.

4.3 Aspects of Fiber Architecture of EHM Patches

4.3.1 Geometric Ventricular Properties

Ellipsoidal Shape

To good approximation the left ventricle can be modeled as a hollow and truncated prolate ellipsoid (depicted in Fig. 4.15) [57, 85, 87, 106]. Most clinical assessments of left ventricular dimensions involve *in vivo* measurements using ultrasound, X-ray or MRI techniques. This means that throughout the measurement process the heart is constantly under pressure, wherefore *in vivo* data has only limited use for accessing left ventricular dimensions of the **unloaded** reference configuration. Obtaining the latter is crucial, since all strains and hence stresses in numerical simulation are based on it (as outlined in Sec. 2.2). As shown in Ref. [107], in addition, widely used MRI measurement techniques show significant deviations from classical autopsy techniques especially for the unloaded excised heart. That said, measurements from different groups and cohorts show only a lose overlap in their results [51, 108, 109].

For the modeling of an idealized elliptical left ventricle, parameters were taken from Ref. [67] as they are in agreement with measurements shown in Ref. [57]. Said parameters can be found in Tab. 4.4.

With the prolate spheroidal coordinates (λ, μ, θ) relating to Euclidian coordinates $\vec{x}$ via

$$
\begin{aligned}
x_1 &= d \cosh \lambda \cos \mu \\
x_2 &= d \sinh \lambda \sin \mu \cos \theta \\
x_3 &= d \sinh \lambda \sin \mu \sin \theta
\end{aligned}
\tag{4.22}
$$

one can define the average over the endocardial surface for any given function f that shows no dependence on θ as

$$
\langle f \rangle_{\mathrm{Surf}} \equiv \frac{2\pi d^2}{A} \int_0^{\pi} f \sinh \lambda \sin \mu \sqrt{\sinh^2 \lambda \cos^2 \mu + \cosh^2 \lambda \sin^2 \mu}\, \mathrm{d}\mu, \tag{4.23}
$$

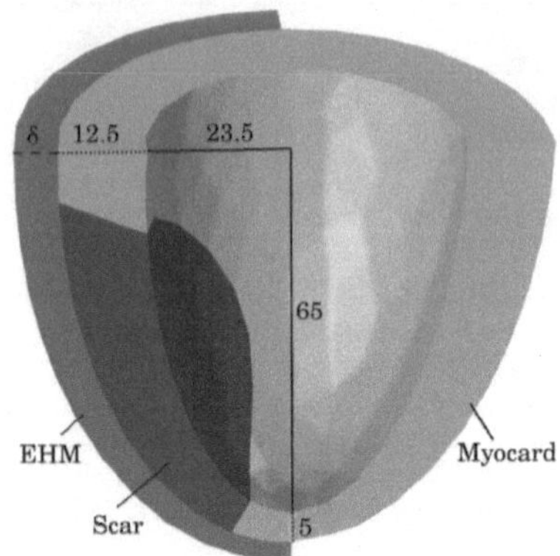

FIGURE 4.15: Dimensions (mm) of the elliptic ventricular geometry corresponding to Tab. 4.4. Colors represent the three different domains EHM patch, scarred tissue and regular myocardium. The thickness of the EHM patch is subject to change between simulation runs. The infarct has a surface area fraction of roughly 20%.

where

$$A = 2\pi \left(a + \frac{c^2}{\sqrt{c^2 - a^2}} \arcsin \frac{\sqrt{c^2 - a^2}}{c} \right) \tag{4.24}$$

is the surface of the ellipse with short and long axis $a = d \sinh \lambda$ and $c = d \cosh \lambda$ respectively. Averaging the relative myocardial wall thickness $\tau(\mu) = |\vec{x}(\lambda_{\text{epi}}) - \vec{x}(\lambda_{\text{endo}})|$ over the endocardial surface, we, thus, obtain

$$\langle \tau / ||\vec{x}(\lambda_{\text{endo}})|| \rangle_{\text{Surf}} = 0.2952. \tag{4.25}$$

This value is in close agreement with the result from a spherical model matched to normalized EDPVR as detailed in Sec. 2.4. Please note that the average in Eq. 4.25 overestimates the actual average wall thickness, since it is not defined as the shortest distance between the endocardial and myocardial surface. The difference between the two definitions, however, is small for the range of parameters used here.

Fiber Architecture

Healthy Left Ventricle: Triggered by the contraction of cardiomyocytes, in a twisting fashion, the heart ejects blood to the vascular system. Cardiomyocytes are cylindrical muscle cells of just roughly 100μm in length and 10-25μm in diameter [110, 111], thus making the acquisition of the cardiac fiber architecture challenging. Yet, this architecture is vital for both structural mechanics and electrophysiology. Even though various efforts have been made over the past decades, the actual fiber architecture still is a vibrant and controversial topic to this date as reviewed in Ref. [7].

In principle, there are two different approaches most frequently used to measure the fiber architecture. It is either diffusion tensor MRI (DT-MRI) [112, 113] or microscopy-based histology [57, 114] that is consulted. While DT-MRI allows fiber mapping of the whole and still intact heart, its resolution does not reach that of microscopy.

Unsurprisingly, in terms of mathematical modeling, there are also several different paths frequently taken. The avenue often used in conjunction with DT-MRI is based on diffeomorphic mapping, where the fiber architecture of a donor's heart is smoothly scaled and deformed to match the geometry of a target heart [73]. This procedure is feasible as long as differences between individuals can be assumed small, which was shown in a cohort of ten individuals by Ref. [75].

Another approach incorporating DT-MRI showing some advances lately is the direct *in vivo* assessment of fiber architecture [11]. Since the data acquisition in DT-MRI is subject to strong time constraints, measurements for the whole heart involve several beating cycles under breath-holding. For some patients, unfortunately, this technique is inadequate as breath-holding can become an insurmountable burden depending on their conditions.

The high resolution of histological data obtained for example from second-harmonic microscopy comes at the cost of the need for accurately prepared tissue specimens. This procedure involves cutting the tissue, therefore releasing residual stresses which might alter the fiber orientation [57]. Additionally, and more importantly, although in principle possible, reconstructing an exhaustive fiber map for the entire heart or even just a single ventricle based on a series of specifically prepared specimens is difficult and time-consuming, rendering it often-times impractical.

The solution to this is a simplification of the data at hand, formulating a single and simple rule describing the myocardial architecture globally. Sparked by the early discoveries of Streeter *et al.* [78], most rule-based methods (RBMs) associate a linear dependency of fiber orientation on tissue depth as depicted in Fig. 4.16. Fibers are assumed to be parallel to the epicardial surface and vary from longitudinal alignment at the endocardium to circumferential alignment at midwall back to a longitudinal alignment at the epicardium.

In summary, it can be noted that diffeomorphic mapping captures a larger amount of details, despite its inferior resolution compared to microscopy, which makes it a more accurate and realistic method in comparison with RBM. However, fiber mapping involves complex registration algorithms and depends heavily on the quality of the donor data, unnecessarily complicating implementations [77]. That said, RBMs are simple to implement, easy to adapt for different shapes and yield good agreement between simulation and experiment in a series of studies [77, 80, 115], wherefore in this work I only make use of them.

For any RBM the need to estimate tissue depth is immanent. A common approach goes back to the work of Potse *et al.* [116], who defined the relative depth at any point in the tissue as

$$e = \frac{d_{\text{endo}}}{d_{\text{endo}} + d_{\text{epi}}}, \tag{4.26}$$

where d_{endo} and d_{epi} denote the minimal distance to endocardium and epicardium respectively. An issue with the definition in Eq. 4.26 is that the minimal distance is not necessarily a regular function, meaning that it can have discontinuities as well as degeneracies, which impede numerical approximations. To overcome the issue of discontinuity in simulation, the authors defined the averaged relative depth $\bar{e}$ which takes into consideration the nearest neighbors in the material mesh. This way, $\nabla\bar{e}$

can be used as a reliable transmural base vector, which later is needed to define the fiber orientation.

Recently, a slightly different myocardial wall depth estimation received an increased interest, as per definition it complies with the regularity condition. *Wong* and *Kuhl* [117] propose a Poisson interpolation scheme which relies on the solution of a homogeneous Laplacian

$$\begin{aligned} &\Delta e = 0, \quad \text{with boundary conditions} \;\; e\big|_{\partial\mathbb{B}_{\text{endo}}} = 0 \;, \;\; e\big|_{\partial\mathbb{B}_{\text{endo}}} = 1 \;, \\ &\text{and} \;\; \mathbf{n}\cdot\nabla e\big|_{\partial\mathbb{B}_{\text{base}}} = 0, \end{aligned} \tag{4.27}$$

where $\partial\mathbb{B}_{\text{endo}}$, $\partial\mathbb{B}_{\text{endo}}$ and $\partial\mathbb{B}_{\text{base}}$ denote endocardial, epicardial and basal surfaces respectively, while $\mathbf{n}$ represents the surface normal vector. This way, a smooth, differentiable and curl free transmural base vector parallel to ∇e emerges. Adapting the approach of Ref. [104], the orthonormal, local, curvilinear base system $(\mathbf{f}, \mathbf{s}, \mathbf{f}\times\mathbf{s})$, as depicted in Fig. 4.16, can be constructed via the algorithm shown in Box 1 below.

1. Define ventricular centerline vector $\mathbf{k}$ along the long axis.
2. Obtain wall depth estimator e by solving Eq. 4.27.
3. Calculate sheet vector via $\mathbf{s} = \nabla e/||\nabla e||$.
4. Calculate fiber vector via $\mathbf{f} = \mathbf{s}\times\mathbf{k}/||\mathbf{s}\times\mathbf{k}||$.
5. Calculate fiber inclination angle $\theta = \theta_{\text{endo}}e + \theta_{\text{epi}}(1-e)$.
6. Rotate fiber vector using Eq. 4.28, s.t. $\mathbf{f} \quad \mathbf{R_s}(\theta)\mathbf{f}$.

(7. Calculate sheet inclination angle $\phi = \phi_{\text{endo}}e + \phi_{\text{epi}}(1-e)$.)

(8. Rotate sheet vector using Eq. 4.28, s.t. $\mathbf{s} \leftarrow \mathbf{R_f}(\phi)\mathbf{s}$.)

Box 1: **Base Construction Algorithm**

The algorithm makes use of the Rodrigues' formula

$$\mathbf{R_x}(\omega) = \begin{pmatrix} \cos\omega + x_1^2 & x_1x_2h - x_3\sin\omega & x_2\sin\omega + x_1x_3h \\ x_3\sin\omega + x_1x_2h & \cos\omega + x_2^2h & -x_1\sin\omega + x_2x_3h \\ -x_2\sin\omega + x_1x_3h & x_1\sin\omega + x_2x_3h & \cos\omega + x_3^2h \end{pmatrix}, \quad \text{with} \;\; h \equiv 1 - \cos\omega, \tag{4.28}$$

which defines a matrix $\mathbf{R_x}(\omega)$ corresponding to a rotation by the angle ω about a normalized vector $\mathbf{x}$. Further, a range for the fiber inclination angles, given by $\theta_{\text{endo}} = 60°$ and $\theta_{\text{epi}} = -60°$ as observed in humans by Ref. [57, 79], is employed. However, this specific choice is not carved in stone. As it has been worked out in Ref. [115], fiber angles strongly influence the EDPVR, leading to an increased VV as $|\theta_{\text{endo}} - \theta_{\text{epi}}|$ increases. In a patient-specific parameterization study [74], it was also found that the maximal fiber angles strongly influence error estimates with best values obtained at $\theta_{\text{endo}} = -\theta_{\text{epi}} = 50°$. Interestingly, though, these findings are contradicted by Niederer *et al.* [45]. They conclude specifically that fiber architecture has so little influence on organ scale metrics that considering patient-specific fiber maps is unnecessary.

In step 5, a linear relation is employed due to its experimental prevalence. However,

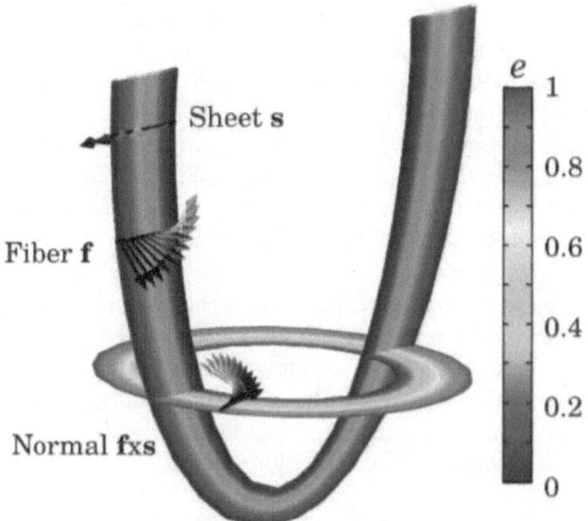

FIGURE 4.16: Ventricular base vectors determined following the algorithm given in Box 1. Variable e is the solution of a Laplace equation according to Eq. 4.27 and measures the local tissue depth. Please note that left- or right-handedness of the base vectors is immaterial.

a cubic law also finds practice in simulations [116], as it shows a better match with experiments performed on dog hearts [78]. The base system constructed here loosely makes use of the assumption that fibers are parallel to the endocardial and epicardial surface, which is justified by the experiments in Ref. [75].

Steps 7 and 8 from the algorithm are only of interest if the constitutive model used is of orthotropic nature (for more details see Sec. 2.2.1). In the literature [80] the values $\phi_{\text{endo}} = 45°$ and $\phi_{\text{epi}} = -45°$ can be found which are based on dog and mouse experiments [76, 118]. However, in Ref. [9] it is pointed out that a different definition for the inclination angle should be used, since, in experiments, it is measured in the longitudinal plane, which resembles the (fs)-plane before step 6 of the algorithm shown in Box 1. This means that instead

$$\phi_{\mathcal{S}} = \arctan(\theta_{\mathcal{S}} \tan \phi'_{\mathcal{S}}) \tag{4.29}$$

with $\phi'_{\text{endo}} = 45°$, $\phi'_{\text{epi}} = -45°$ and $\mathcal{S} \in \{\text{endo, epi}\}$ is proposed. The organization of the sheets is delicate to compute as discussed by *Gilbert et al.* [119]. As it varies strongly between different sections of the ventricle [77, 111] and displays irregular angle flips on a submillimeter scale [119], wherefore precise numbers have to be taken with care. For a HO model, though, it has been shown that variability in sheet orientation only shows little impact on stress development in the left ventricle [76]. Since fiber dispersion reduces directional sensitivity as shown in Ref. [49], it is reasonable that also for the 2SGST model sheet direction plays a minor role. That said, a transmural variation of sheet orientation is omitted in the simulations presented below. Instead, the values $\phi_{\text{endo}} = \phi_{\text{epi}} = 0$ are used. For the dispersion coefficients for fibers and sheets respectively I adopt the values $b_{\rho_{\text{f}}} = 4.5$ and $b_{\rho_{\text{s}}} = 3.9$ which were obtained from human myocardium [57].

Infarct: In Sec. 1.2 the different phases of tissue remodeling are mentioned. This remodeling encompasses not only an increase in local stiffness, particularly in fiber direction but also a change in fiber orientation. Where cardiomyocytes die and get replaced by collagen fibers, these reorient such that they maximize their load-bearing capacity, meaning that they point in the direction of principal strain [120]. For a scar at the free wall as depicted in Fig. 4.15, this implicates a predominantly circumferentially alignment [28, 121]. In contrast, at the apex, strains are distributed more broadly and so are collagen fibers. This is the reason, why, for the scar, I choose the values $\theta_{\text{endo}} = \theta_{\text{epi}} = \phi_{\text{endo}} = \phi_{\text{epi}} = 0$.

Along with the mean fiber orientation, of course, also the dispersion of the collagen is different from that of the myocytes. However, to my knowledge, there exists currently no study which quantifies fiber dispersion in infarcted myocardium. Therefore, and in an effort to stay in line with the simplifications introduced for the spherical model, the dispersion for the scarred tissue is assumed to be identical to that of healthy myocardium as defined in the previous section.

EHM patch: In Ref. [122] it has been shown that anisotropic reinforcement of infarcts can improve pump function. In particular, longitudinal reinforcement was shown to be superior over circumferential reinforcement. This sparks the question of whether and how in an EHM patch its performance is influenced by the fiber architecture. While, just like the scarred tissue, in simulation EHM is considered to display the same dispersion as healthy myocardium, three different cases for the mean fiber orientation are assumed. The first two cases revolve around the assumption that it is possible to train EHM patches prior to implantation, demanding a maturation, which, as discussed in Sec. 1.3, entails considerable complications [40]. Just as in Ref. [122], these two cases comprise longitudinal and circumferential mean fiber alignment as displayed in Fig. 4.17. The third case comprises remodeling occurring after implantation happened. While it is still unclear how fibers effectively change their alignment, it is postulated here that they align smoothly with the surrounding healthy tissue. This is realized through solving the Laplace equation for the individual base vectors with Dirichlet BCs such that the base system, there, is continuous. A subsequent Gram-Schmidt process ensures that the base vectors are be orthonormal.

4.3.2 Boundary Conditions

The Heart is engulfed in the pericardium, surrounded by the lungs, stomach, and diaphragm, all pressuring it from the outside, while the pulmonary artery supplies the heart with freshly oxygenized blood, thus elevating the interior blood pressure. In preparation to render computational simulations possible, it is obligatory to reduce the complexity of this zoo of different boundary conditions in a confined manner. Considering that I do not intend to simulate the fluid dynamics of the blood I have to replace the fluid-structure interaction at the endocardium with a suitable boundary condition (BC). It is judicious to assign a homogeneous pressure, with zero value at early diastole versus 8-12 mmHg [61, 73] EDP and values around 100 mmHg at the end of systole.

Monoventricular, just like biventricular, models commonly content themselves with the assumption of a free outer wall, hence rendering its surrounding devoid. However, studies incorporating the pericardium, a slippery sack enveloping and thereby stabilizing almost the entire heart (see Fig. 1.1), showed that it strongly influences cardiac mechanics [100, 123, 134, 135]. While the *in vivo* parameter estimation using DT-MRI strain measurements yields good agreement between experiment and simulation

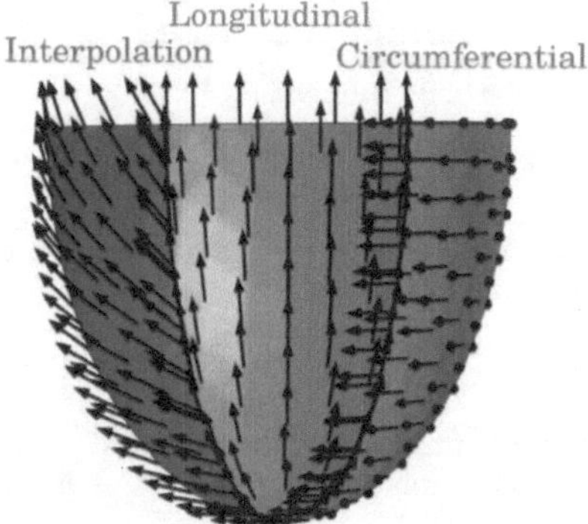

FIGURE 4.17: EHM patch with the three distinct mean fiber alignments corresponding to different simulations as shown in Fig. 4.20. Circumferential and longitudinal alignments are based on the postulate that tissue entrainment prior to implantation is possible. Smooth interpolation of the base belonging to the surrounding healthy tissue reflects remodeling after implantation. Fiber orientation exerts only little transmural variation which is why only fibers on the surface are shown.

concerning the EF, the deformation patterns showed much stronger accordance to imaging data after a spring like representation of the pericardium was included. Yet, also these models leave the effect of external organs to wonder. For simplicity, the epicardium is chosen to be an open boundary.

The left atrium is connected to the left ventricle via the mitral valve, which in turn is surrounded by a fibrous ring known as the mitral annulus. The geometry presented in Fig 4.15 is truncated at the interface between the mitral annulus and the myocardium (c.f. Fig 1.1). Although this truncation is frequently used, it is still rather artificial, traversing fibroelastic connective tissue, thus giving rise to complex BCs at the base. In order to make the interface numerically tractable nonetheless, strong simplifications are made. The collagenous material, the mitral annulus is made of, is rather stiff, which can be accounted for by applying rigid BCs [70]. Compared with experimental results, however, this appears to be an oversimplification [123]. Finding the right amount of complexity is not an easy task – Circumstances fertilizing scientific creativity.

In Tab. 4.5 prominent BCs are listed and briefly described, several of which can be represented using a spring foundation. Therein, the first Piola-Kirchoff stress $\mathbf{P}$ is balanced on the boundary via

$$\mathbf{Pn} = [\nu_r \mathbf{e}_r \otimes \mathbf{e}_r + \nu_z \mathbf{e}_z \otimes \mathbf{e}_z + \nu_\phi \mathbf{e}_\phi \otimes \mathbf{e}_\phi] (\mathbf{u} - \mathbf{u}_0), \tag{4.30}$$

where $\mathbf{e}_r, \mathbf{e}_z$, and $\mathbf{e}_\phi$ are the radial, longitudinal, and circumferential base vectors respectively in cylindrical coordinates while $\mathbf{u}$ describes the local displacement at the basal boundary. The reference displacement $\mathbf{u}_0$ can be determined by experimental data but often-times it is simply set equal to zero. The spring constants ν_r, ν_z, and ν_ϕ typically are rather large, resembling the stiffness of the mitral annulus. For example in Ref. [104, 123] the value $\nu_r = \nu_z = \nu_\phi = 50\,\mathrm{kPa/cm}$ is used, allowing only

Description	Ref.
The base is held completely fixed in all directions.	[70]
The base surface is kept fixed in accordance with experimentally derived data.	[47]
Translation along and rotation about longitudinal axis are forbidden, while radial stretching still is allowed.	[67, 73, 98, 115]
Only either the outer or inner ring of the base surface are held fixed, while the rest may deform unconstrained.	[45, 118]
A spring foundation aligns simulation with experiment, while at the same time reducing influence of experimental errors and discontinuities.	[104, 123]
Longitudinal displacement is constrained and in plane deformation is restricted with a spring foundation	[100]
Only the center of mass is kept fixed. It is unclear how rotation is penalized.	[60]

TABLE 4.5: Short summary of some common base plane BCs. Not only are the fromalisms and the emanating algorithms different but also the biology that is hence captured. A clear recepe of when to use which formalism remains disguised . For more details please see Ref. [59].

for small deformations at the base including translation in the long-axis direction. The geometry outlined in Sec. 4.3.1 represents a ventricle which is not directly cut underneath the mitral annulus and instead has its base at its largest extent in the short-axis plane. With the intention not to undercut the pump volume of the heart in the simulations below I employ rather soft BCs as done in Ref. [100]. They use Eq. 4.30 with the values

$$\nu_z = \infty, \qquad \nu_r = \nu_\phi = 0.5\,\mathrm{kPa/cm} \qquad \text{and} \qquad \mathbf{u}_0 = 0, \tag{4.31}$$

thus completely denying out of plane movement while twist and radial displacement still is allowed. A positive side effect of using such a spring foundation is that, contrary to a fixed boundary, peak stresses get reduced thanks to the additional degree of freedom. As discussed in Ref. [49], otherwise, internal angles can get so small that evaluating derivatives proves difficult at the edges, which, in turn, affects the accuracy and convergence of the FEM solver. Although the EHM patch shares the basal boundary, it is not directly connected to the structure of the mitral annulus, which is why a free BC is chosen instead.

4.3.3 Constitutive parameters

For the studies conducted in Sec. 4.2 an isotropic constitutive law is used, which only comprises three parameters, therefore allowing for a single curve -the Klotz curve in this case- to be used as a reliable reference. Nonetheless, the fitting procedure is accompanied by large ambiguities in the choice for the fit parameters, which, in parts, explains the large fitting errors (see Tab. 2.2). When analyzing the influence of the fiber architecture, it is important, not only to capture it in the contractile law as

	a	b	a_f	b_f	a_s	b_s	a_{fs}	b_{fs}	b_{ρ_f}	b_{ρ_s}
Simple Shear	0.784	7.08	1.64	10.5	0.53	8.9	0	—	4.5	3.9
Biaxial Stretch	1.01	22.5	1.43	47.5	—	—	—	—		

TABLE 4.6: Fit parameters for the 2SGST model corresponding to the plots shown in Fig. 4.18 together with the predefined fiber and sheet dispersion coefficients b_{ρ_f} and b_{ρ_s}. Interestingly, although set as a free parameter in case of simple shear, the coupling coefficient a_{fs} reached zero after optimization, indicating the capacity of dispersion to capture fiber-sheet coupling.

defined in Eq. 4.11b, but also to consider it in the passive material law, specifically when treating the purely passive scarred tissue. For that purpose, I use a 2SGST adaption of the HO model (see Sec. 2.2.1), which gives rise to eight passive material parameters. As previously demonstrated for the dispersion-free HO model in Fig. 2.3, these parameters are optimized using a minimum chi-square estimation and simple shear data from experiments performed on human cardiac tissue by Sommer *et al.* [57]. The same model is also used to fit biaxial extension tests with the little adjustment that sheet and coupling terms are neglected. The resultant fits alongside the resultant optimized parameters are shown in Fig. 4.18.

The circumstance that the two different data sets show strongly differing stiffnesses albeit originating from the same species[2] is a concern not only faced in my analysis. It is also addressed by Gütlekin *et al.* [67], who use a viscoelastic 0GST model to describe the data. Needless to say that they did not succeed in describing both data sets with a single fit. It is, to this date, unclear whether this shortcoming is to be addressed by a change in constitutive models or whether the experimental setup, by design, does not allow for a comparison. Possibly, the fact that the tissue slabs used for biaxial extension tests are much larger than the cubes used for simple shear renders the two setups incompatible, or maybe tissue softening has to be taken into account on a model level. In a preceding analysis (not shown), I used fiber dispersion to different degrees with the hope the explain the experimental data but even the AI could not match simple shear and biaxial extension simultaneously.

The question yet left to answer is which of the two data sets appears more trustworthy. Since in simulation the EDV proves to be unreasonably small in the case of biaxial stretch data (103 mL vs. 124 mL), plus the fact that the resultant Klotz curve deviates more strongly from the best fit of the spherical model (see Sec. 4.18d), I choose to use the results obtained from simple shear data in subsequent simulations.

Still, these parameters paired with the geometry defined in Sec. 4.3.1 entail a rather stiff ventricle, demanding contractions close to the minimal sarcomere length λ_0 (c.f. 4.5). Therefore, and as a means to keep the Ees at reasonable levels, I choose to adjust the contractile parameter T_a such that an EF of 60% is met[3]. This leads to T_a = 950 kPa entailing an Ees of 7.88 mmHg/mL which compares nicely to the literature (see Sec. 1.1.2) although it still is a comparably large value.

[2]We were also supplied with experimental data from a single individual and still faced the same issue.

[3]This contrasts the choice of EF=66% previously made in Sec. 4.2.

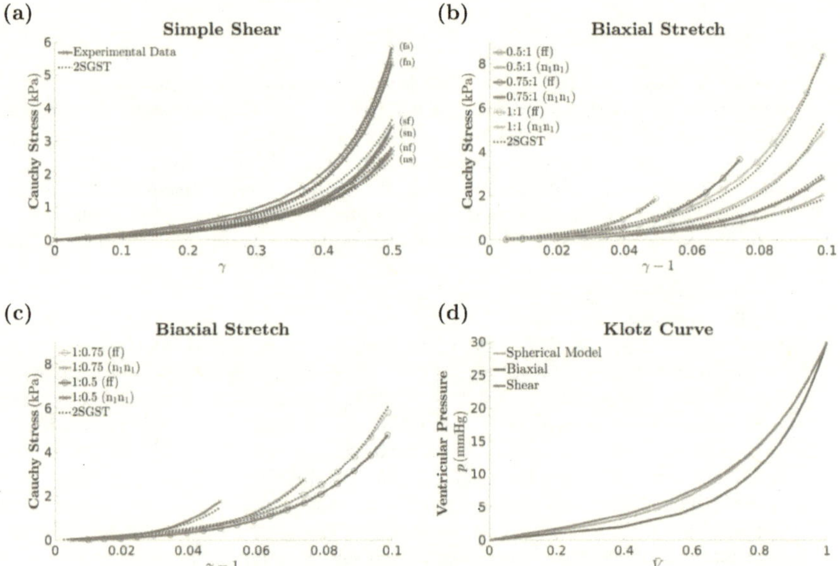

FIGURE 4.18: Optimization of the 2SGST adaption of Eq. 2.22 to experimental data taken from Ref. [57]. (a) and (b) Biaxial stretch data split into two subplots for better readability. Although both data sets are nicely fit, simple shear and biaxial stretch express strong deviations concerning the optimal parameters. Biaxial stretch data displays much larger stiffening coefficients b and b_f yielding much smaller EDV in simulation. The biaxial stretch data also leads to a larger deviation from the spherical model fit to the Klotz data (see Sec. 2.4) wherefore I choose to use the simple shear data for the study instead. The corresponding fit parameters can be found in Tab. 4.6.

4.3.4 Results

With the geometry, fiber architecture, boundary conditions, passive and active materials described in the previous sections, the simulation almost can be carried out. Only the constitutive law for the scar is left to be determined. In an identical manner as in Sec. 4.2, it is defined to share the same passive model parameters as the healthy myocardium just furnished with a factor

$$\Psi_{\text{inf}} = \alpha \Psi^{\text{2SGST}}_{\text{healthy}} \tag{4.32}$$

integrating apparent material softening. Since the analysis of the spherical model did not entail qualitative differences based on the value of the factor it will remain $\alpha = 1/2$ throughout the entire investigation.

Similar to the findings in Sec. 4.2, neither infarction nor grafting an EHM patch on the scar shows any relevant influence on the EDPVR which is presented in Fig. 4.19a. This is contrasted by the ESPVR. Infarction, of course, heavily impairs pump function illustrated by a drop from 60% to 35% in EF depicted in Fig. 4.19c. In all cases, the pump function greatly benefits from the addition of EHM patches. What comes to a huge surprise, though, is how little it depends on the actual thickness fraction δ of the EHM (here calculated with respect to the myocardial wall thickness at the base τ). This conflicts previous results shown in Fig. 4.10c. Using Eq. 4.25 it is possible to translate the thickness fractions of the elliptical model to those of the spherical model, resulting in

$$\delta: \qquad 1/4 \rightarrow 0.057 \qquad 1/3 \rightarrow 0.077 \qquad 1/2 \rightarrow 0.116. \tag{4.33}$$

Now, considering $\delta = 0.05$ and $\delta = 0.1$ with $\theta = 180°$ in the spherical model involves an increase in EF by more than 5 percentage points (pp), whereas in the elliptical model increasing the patch thickness by a twofold is accompanied by a respective increase in EF of 2 pp at most, which is achieved in the case of circumferential alignment. Variation between the different fiber alignments is slightly larger with a difference of 4 pp between longitudinal and interpolated fibers at $\delta = 1/4$. Interestingly, the interpolated fiber alignment, which is meant to reflect remodeling in the EHM and falls in between longitudinal and circumferential alignment (see Fig. 4.17), shows the weakest increase in EF. Considering Ees on the other hand, the interpolated fiber architecture indeed lies in between the two extremal arrangements. As shown in Fig. 4.19b, the longitudinal alignment has the strongest potential of recovery, whereas circumferential alignment performs even worse than the infarct alone, thus shattering the intuition that more muscle tissue should yield stronger contractile performance. This intuition, however, holds only as long as the additional tissue works conjoined with the tissue already present. Thus, it can be concluded that, at least in parts, the cardiomyocytes in circumferential alignment work against those in the healthy tissue. Similar to the spherical model, the Ees of the circumferential alignment shows practically no dependents on patch thickness. This is contrasted by the other two alignments, thus highlighting the importance to study realistic fiber arrangements.

Different fiber alignments impact how contraction alters the shape of the left ventricle. In Fig. 4.20 it can be observed that a longitudinal arrangement, expectedly, leads to shortening along the long axis, whereas the other two arrangements produce rather elongated shapes. The von Mises stress (see Eq. 25 in Ref. [49]) in the border zone of the infarct, also depicted in Fig. 4.20, shows the overall smallest values for the longitudinal alignment. As discussed in Sec. 1.2, reducing the border zone stresses

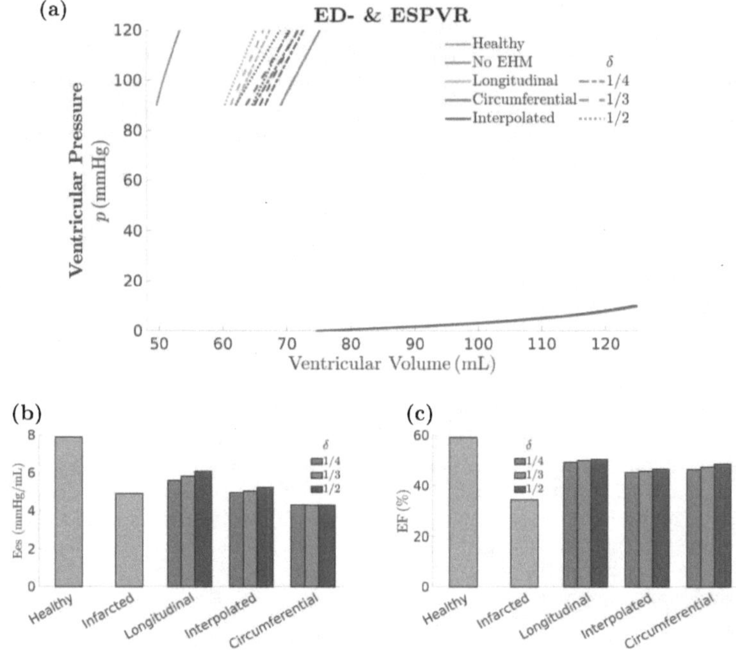

FIGURE 4.19: (a) EDPVR and ESPVR for different fiber orientations and patch thickness fractions δ (relative to τ) indicated by the gray colored legend entries. The EDPVR shows virtually no dependence on either fiber orientation wherefore the resultant curves overlap almost perfectly. In contrast, the ESPVR is heavily influenced by both. (b) Ees corresponding to (a). How much it changes for different values of θ depends on the fiber architecture. (c) Resultant EF. Although the effects are small, the longitudinal arrangement shows best Ees and EF recoveries.

likely reduces the risk for infarct growth, which favors longitudinal alignment over the others. For similar reasons it is conceivable that stresses and their gradient should be kept small at the interface between scar and EHM. In Fig. 4.21 the von Mises stress along the cut line depicted in Fig. 4.20 can be examined. Increasing the wall thickness eases cooperation between ventricle and EHM by reducing absolute wall stresses at the interface. Smallest stress values and smallest gradients belong to the interpolated base system directly followed by the longitudinal alignment.

4.3.5 Conclusion & Discussion

In this section, I reviewed current approaches in computational simulations of the left ventricle entailing BCs and fiber architecture, which I adjusted to cope with the simplistic spherical model from Sec. 4.2.2. Of course, these choices strongly affect the entire analysis, and specifically so the numeric values. For example a base BC weighting the stiffness of the mitral annulus more strongly would necessitate even stronger

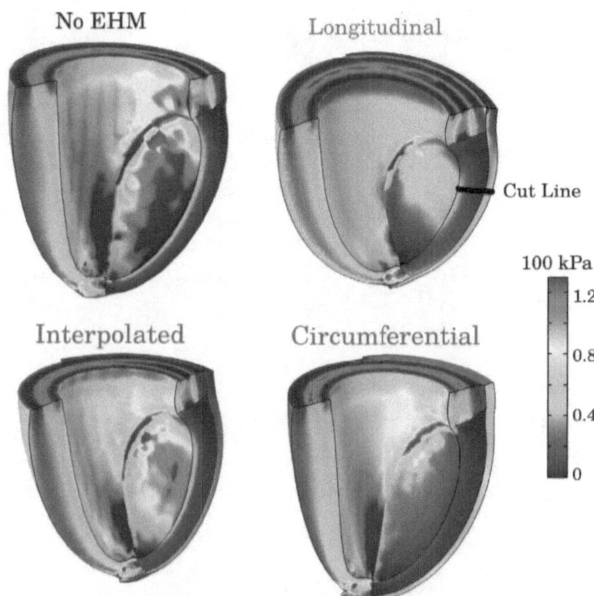

FIGURE 4.20: Shapes and the von Mises Stress (Eq. 25 Ref. [49]) of the ventricle at the end of systole for the various fiber architectures of the EHM patch at a thickness $\delta = 1/2$ as shown in Fig. 4.17. In all cases, reduced von Mises stresses compared to the case of no EHM graft are reported in the border zone, with the overall smallest values observed for the longitudinal alignment. Along the *cut line* von Mises stresses are the smallest for the interpolated base system as presented in Fig. 4.21.

contractile forces, which, in turn, alters how infarct and EHM interact. That said, although the attempt was made to include as realistic material properties as possible derived from human and animal experiments likewise, a quantitative conclusion based on my simulations is impermissible. And although the strength of these simulations is not the accurate prediction of turnout EF or Ees, qualitative trends are clearly visible.

The great advantage of grafts made of active biomaterial is clearly highlighted in the different pressure-volume relation. Almost no changes are observed during diastole, allowing for maximal inflation while systolic contraction negates bulging and supports the border zone material, thus increasing the ejected blood volume. From Fig. 4.19c it becomes evident that these effects dominate over fiber architecture and it can be assumed that even an EHM with purely randomly distributed fibers, bare of any mean fiber direction, promotes a considerable increase in cardiac pump function.

Yet, if fiber directions are explicitly considered, while not excelling in any particular field by any stretch of the definition, the longitudinal alignment shows improvement in EF and Ees over the alternatives, which is in agreement with the findings described in Refs. [121, 122] where the effects of non-bilogical, noncontractile, anistropic reinforecement of scarred tissue were tested.

In order to support these findings, additional simulations, covering a larger range

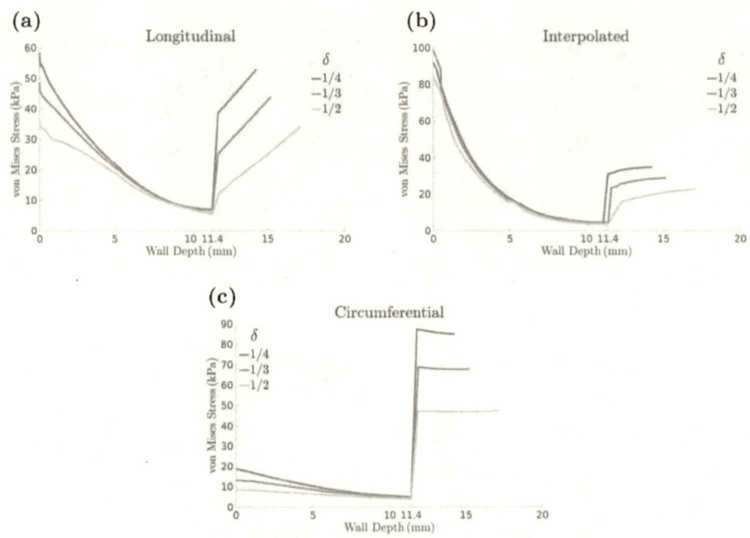

FIGURE 4.21: Transmural von Mises stresses along the cut line depicted in Fig. 4.20. In all cases it can be observed that, as EHM thickness δ increases, the stresses decline. Along the cut line the scar exhibits a depth of roughly 11.4 mm. This is the spot where stresses show sudden jumps. Here the interpolated fiber architecture shows smallest absolute values and smallest gradients directly followed by the longitudinal arrangement.

of parameters, are mandatory. A possible approach could be the consultation of machine learning which would allow probing also quantitative effects while, at the same time, providing a measure of accuracy. Problematic with such an approach is to find reasonable bounds for the parameter space as not all combinations of passive and active material properties have real-life relevance. This was, for example, the reasoning behind discarding human biaxial stretch data, as it did not show desirable EDVs and did not comply with the Klotz curve. When inquiring a larger parameter space additional arbiters must be installed to ensure relevance.

The mere fact that, to this date, there is no constitutive model which can match biaxial and simple shear data of the same heart simultaneously challenges both, experiment and mathematical description. Still, even a model is found to be trustworthy and the parameters derived from average human data and combine it with the average geometry of the LV using average fiber and sheet architectures together with average rest sarcomere length and adjusted contractile force to capture the average EF, there is no guaranty that the result yields the average values for the EDPVR and ESPVR. This ambiguity is due to the complex, nonlinear, and intertwined interaction between all constituents principally prohibiting the connection between separately obtained averages. A potential bypass to this issue are patients specific models where passive and active material properties are not adopted to *ex vivo* but rather *in vivo* experimental data involving, for example, MRI. Such measurements, expectedly, carry their own disadvantages like for example the infidelity of DT-MRI derived fiber architectures. Another issue poses the reference configuration which, due to external loads, never is captured throughout a beating cycle. The amount of information obtained through MRI strain and volume measurements is so scarce that only heavily reduced constitutive models can be matched adequately, thus compromising their ability to extrapolate the impact of EHM. In a perfect world, the methods laid out in this work would be tested against both, *ex vivo* and *in vivo* experiments of individual humans before and after implantation of EHM, which, all things considered, will remain unfeasible in the near future.

Particular attention appertains to the validity of the active contractile law considering transversely isotropic like orthotropic representation introduced in Sec. 4.1. The counterparts to Eq. 4.11b, found in the literature presented, are based on *ex vivo* stress-strain curves of sarcomeres and were tested in simulations against *in vivo* whole heart/ventricle experiments, whereas the intermittent tissue level, to my knowledge, is omitted. Thus an important issue is plainly neglected which is the compatibility between active and passive material laws on said tissue level. If two different experimental protocols targeting passive tissue response, i.e. biaxial stretch and simple shear, are incompatible, how can we safely assume that it should hold between diastole and systole? The problem cements when considering that force-length relationships typically (if not all) are performed with a monoaxial setup despite the fact that systole also involves strong shearing. In addition, it became popular recently to neglect energy terms in the constitutive law associated with fibers under compression [64, 83, 124]. This is reasonable, as fibers are slim and buckle easily. Especially for collagen and hence scarred tissue it is suggested in future studies to account and check for the effect of compression of fibers. Within the framework of *COMSOL*, to the best of my knowledge, this approach remains impractical, considering that *COMSOL* only allows for differentiable strain energy densities to be used.

Another improvement could be achieved through adaption of BCs. Dealing with only the left ventricle prompts the question of whether excluding the atria and the right ventricle can be justified in a quantitative analysis. After all, in Refs. [45, 115] the importance of the right ventricle (RV) on the EDPVR was demonstrated as it could increase the VV by up to 5% at a ventricular pressure of 10 mmHg.

www.ingramcontent.com/pod-product-compliance
Lightning Source LLC
LaVergne TN
LVHW040909150826
845672LV00007B/1964

* 9 7 8 3 3 8 4 2 1 3 4 9 5 *